Progressive Health Care Management Strategies

Donald N. Lombardi, Ph.D.

AHA books are published by
American Hospital Publishing, Inc.,
an American Hospital Association company

Library of Congress Cataloging-in-Publication Data

Lombardi, Donald N., 1956–
    Progressive health care management strategies / Donald N. Lombardi.
        p.   cm.
    Includes bibliographical references.
    ISBN 1-55648-092-X (pbk.)
    1. Health services administration.   I. Title.
    [DNLM: 1. Health Facility Administrators—organization & administration.   2. Staff Development—methods.   WX 159 L842P]
    RA971.L65   1992
    362.1'1'068—dc20
    DNLM/DLC
    for Library of Congress   92-49632
                                                                         CIP

Catalog no. 088300

©1992 by American Hospital Publishing, Inc.,
an American Hospital Association company

Printed in the USA

𝔸𝕙𝔸 is a service mark of the American Hospital Association used under license by American Hospital Publishing, Inc.

Text set in Palatino
3M—09/92—0325

Richard Hill, Project Editor
Teresa Cappetta-Kroger, Production Editor
Marcia Bottoms, Managing Editor
Peggy DuMais, Production Coordinator
Cheryl Kusek, Cover Designer
Brian Schenk, Books Division Director

To Deborah Ann

Contents

About the Author

Donald N. Lombardi, Ph.D., is the principal partner of CHR/InterVista, Inc., a health care human resources consulting firm headquartered in Hackettstown, New Jersey. He has designed and implemented human resources systems in more than 100 health care organizations and holds more than 50 copyrights on human resources and industrial psychology management systems and programs. Prior to undertaking his consulting work, Dr. Lombardi held top personnel positions with American Hospital Supply Corporation and with Bristol-Myers, where he was instrumental in innovating and installing management systems in the company's North American, Caribbean, and European operations.

As an officer in the U.S. Marine Corps, Dr. Lombardi designed several educational and manpower management programs that were adopted for use throughout the entire range of armed forces personnel and were lauded by both civilian and military experts. He has written numerous articles for publications ranging from *Philadelphia Magazine* to *Administrative Radiology*. His books include *Handbook of Personnel Selection and Performance Evaluation in Healthcare* and *Stress and the Healthcare Environment*, both considered the definitive texts in their subject areas.

Dr. Lombardi is also a faculty member of the Graduate School of Public Administration of Seton Hall University in South Orange, New Jersey, and he teaches three accreditation courses for the American College of Healthcare Executives.

List of Figures and Tables

Preface

Few professions face the formidable challenges with which health care managers and executives are confronted in this decade. Mounting public scrutiny, widespread consumer pessimism, and increasing governmental interaction with the health care community all contribute to a confluence of uncertainty and apprehension. At the center of the turmoil is the health care manager, the individual charged with bringing together diverse talents and various resources within the organization. The health care manager must formulate a progressive strategy to ensure that the organization not only survives but *thrives* in a tumultuous business arena.

Progressive Health Care Management Strategies is intended to be a handbook for the health care management professional in these turbulent times. With its practical approaches and proven techniques, the book serves as a pragmatic reference on systems and strategies utilized by professionals throughout the field. The book is supportive of organizational theory and management principles, but its goal is to give each reader the realistic and readily usable applications that will optimize his or her effectiveness in carrying out a manager's responsibilities and the organization's mission.

The focus of the entire book is *progressive management*, a term that encompasses both the successful management of today's activities and, perhaps more important, of tomorrow's challenges. The discussion of progressive management is treated in two parts. Part one, "The Progressive Health Care Manager," examines the role of the effective health care manager and provides dozens of strategies that can be utilized immediately by a manager at any level of the organization. This part allows each reader to focus on the management of human resources (including staff professionals) at his or her particular facility. Furthermore, the six chapters constituting part one examine specific situations that confront the manager frequently and delineate methods for achieving the highest level of employee performance even in the most difficult circumstances.

Part two, "The Progressive Health Care Organization," reviews not only the line management but also the organizationwide aspects of progressive health care management. In other words, this part of the book widens the scope of the discussion to serve the particular needs of middle and senior managers and executives, as well as the needs of line managers and supervisors who aspire to fill those administrative positions some day.

The "value-driven" strategies woven throughout the book are further illumined in part two with two case studies, each providing an array of examples and innovative methods of implementation. The utilization of these strategies—which have been proven effective by their successful use at leading health care organizations—can provide readers with a foundation for learning to thrive in what is certain to be the most uncertain period of modern health care management.

Each of the five appendixes at the end of the book offers a foundational tool for developing a methodology that promotes workplace behaviors that reflect an organization's mission and goals. Appendix A sets out 20 desirable organizational values (based on chapter 3) and presents 100 questions for interviewing prospective employees or managers. Appendix B presents a model performance evaluation plan that numerically scores employees on goal attainment and also on their commitment to organizational values. Appendix C lists 50 sample motivators in five key areas (based on chapter 4). Appendix D lists 20 strategies and gives 60 possible methods of implementation (based on chapter 7). Appendix E provides 10 customer community strategies and 10 organizational business strategies for implementation.

In total, *Progressive Health Care Management Strategies* gives the reader at least one resource for managing people and situations in the health care setting to ensure the progressive development of every member of the team. As a reference, the book provides a framework for taking effective management action on a day-to-day basis. As a handbook, it makes "real" the themes and strategies that managers often hear are vital to garnering optimal staff performance. Finally, as a guide it can contribute toward making the health care workplace a progressive custodian of the public trust—which, after all, is health care's most basic charter.

Acknowledgments

This book, as well as all of my work, is an extension of my wife's patient and unwavering support, and thus is rightly dedicated to her. My parents also deserve a tremendous amount of credit. I hope that my work justifies all the trips to the library my mother embarked on during my youth, and I hope it reflects the insightful "value-driven" guidance I received from my father. In addition, my two uncles—one a noted Jesuit educator and one a Marine colonel—certainly have been more than role models, and my grandparents, brothers, cousins, in-laws, and friends have all inspired any worthwhile work I produce. Last but not least, I want to say a special word of thanks to Rick Hill, project editor at American Hospital Publishing, for his encouragement and exemplary effort in shaping and editing this book.

Part One

The Progressive Health Care Manager

Chapter 1

The Need for Progressive Strategies

The current age of health care is a period marked by ultracompetitiveness, alternative delivery systems, shrinking resources, and increased public scrutiny. The difference between the successful organization and the "also-ran" or failing institution will be intelligent progressive management from the board and the CEO to the first-line supervisors. The premier health care manager of the 1990s is the one who skillfully incorporates ethical standards, progressive people management, and innovative leadership strategies into a winning approach for optimum efficiency and maximum effectiveness.

A series of studies published in recent years has expounded severe consequences for the health care organization that does not rise to the increasing challenges of this unique business setting. The most accepted study, the Delphi study compiled by Arthur Andersen & Company in 1991, suggests that in excess of 900 health care institutions will have gone out of business or have been absorbed by larger organizations by the year 2000.[1] To avoid being included in this statistic, the successful health care organization must ensure that all of its managerial staff provide a style of leadership that is ethically sound; a managerial approach that is insightful and resourceful; and an organizational management system that makes optimum use of all operational resources, financial resources, and—perhaps most important—human resources. As the health care customer community becomes even more circumspect and demanding in seeking excellence in health care, the difference between an institution that truly serves its customer/patient and one that falls by the wayside will be determined by the quality of individual managers and their ability to artfully maximize their business responsibilities.

In essence, *progressive health care management* is the artful incorporation of three components serving as the basis for the daily activities and decisions of managers:

- *Organizational ethics:* Managers must bring to the workplace sound, value-driven behavioral norms that they seek to instill in their staff and apply to all business dealings.
- *People management skills:* Managers must demonstrate sound human resources practices throughout the organization that encourage maximum input and output from each employee.
- *Leadership skills:* Managers must bring clear vision and stellar business standards to their jobs each day that lead to decisive action and an orientation toward community service.

This chapter addresses each of these three components; later chapters introduce proven strategies that managers and executives can use to ensure progressive health care management.

☐ Organizational Ethics

The influence of sound organizational ethics stems from the re-emergence of business ethics as a national issue, which has important ramifications for health care managers and professionals throughout the field.

Ethics and the Health Care Customer Community

The provision of health care services is an activity that plays a prominent part in the life of every American consumer, and health care providers are always a constant presence in communities throughout the nation. Seen as a public trust, a needed provider, and a source of immediate remedy in the most critical times in a person's life, the health care organization naturally is held to the highest standards of ethical conduct and optimum performance. Within a local community—whether rural, suburban, or urban—the health care provider (although not part of the local government hierarchy) is deemed as important as the police force, fire squad, or school system. Because of the delicate nature of its service provision, its profound impact on a person's life and life-style, and its permanent effect, the health care business naturally falls under more intense quality assessment by the customer/patient; more than would a hamburger joint or a clothing store, for example. With the increased attention toward ethical business standards, the health care organization now finds itself under even greater pressure to "do the right thing" in every given situation.

The national perception of health care has contributed to this increased pressure. As Americans become aware of the nursing shortage and other situations that could adversely affect the quality of health care (overcrowded emergency rooms, lack of large city municipal health care providers, and financial shortages across the field), a suspicion has grown nationally about the basic competence of health care organizations. Additionally, the American consumer, conditioned to believe that everything is better in this country, is now faced with information that indicates that countries in Scandinavia and Western Europe indeed have better health care systems. Politicians such as Senator Edward Kennedy of Massachusetts are currently advocating national health care systems that are similar to those in Germany, Sweden, and Canada. As Americans become increasingly aware of this country's homeless and the growing underclass, the need for a national health care system seems to emerging as a popular cause.

Implicit in this desire for a national health care system is the perception that a national health system would ensure a national standard of health care quality. Doubts about the competence of local community hospitals are fed as the six o'clock news reports malpractice cases, closing facilities, and the skyrocketing cost of health insurance. Most issues of concern to the health care customer/patient have ethical implications of one sort or another.

In a recent seminar for the American College of Healthcare Executives (ACHE), a top administrator of a Pennsylvania hospital made a comment that perhaps illustrates the relationship between the general current perception of health care and its relationship to ethical standards in health care management. He said, "Fifteen years ago, the health care organization, and the individuals who ran the facility, was seen as the good guys. Now, not only are we not seen as the good guys, but we are perhaps seen as persons who are taking advantage of a favorable supply/demand situation at the expense of people's well-being."

This "bad guy" perception is rooted in several factors that are related to ethical issues. The increase in malpractice lawsuits, for example, is often seen by the public as being a result of decisions made in hospital environments. After all, the hospitals hire the physicians, allow them to practice, and ostensibly facilitate the circumstances in which the malpractice can occur. If the hospital managers were truly ethical, they would be more demanding and attentive to physicians' actions and malpractice would not be prominent—or so the popular reasoning goes. Most health care managers would agree that, because of a number of factors beyond their control, this popular reasoning is somewhat invalid. The fact remains, however, that strong ethical action must be taken in every regard in physician relationships and in the portrayal of sound medical competence to the customer/patient community.

In another vein, consider the media's current fascination with health care at both the local and national levels. Recently, the author's firm conducted a major outplacement project in upstate New York. This involved the very ethical action of a major health care provider in a small city that contracted outplacement services so that employees terminated due to the hospital's financial trouble could readily find other employment. The financial trouble suffered by this hospital was due primarily to the city's widescale employment situation and lack of opportunity at the local production mills, which has plagued many northern cities in recent times due to migration to the Southwest as well as foreign pervasion of the manufacturing field. Clearly, the hospital was not responsible for the circumstances leading to the termination, nor was it unethical in terminating these employees. However, the local media, including the television station, two town newspapers, and a radio station, chose to report the termination procedure and the layoff as big news. Although the provision of outplacement services was a very positive action taken by the hospital, viewers may have been given a much different impression. From the thread of a local hospital's problems, one reporter wove a summary of the status of health care in America.

Another media fascination concerns the profitability of insurance providers and the increased cost of insurance to the typical American. It is perhaps a common perception that health care providers and insurance companies work together to raise costs and yet provide fewer services. The deductible for many insurance companies has risen by large percentages in recent years, and a response among several insurance providers is to offer clients a product called "flex benefits." In effect, *flex benefits* allow employees to select from their employers' insurance policy only the coverage they need, thus allaying cost of coverage their spouse might have, or what they receive from other sources, or perhaps coverage they do not need. This "menu-type" approach to insurance reflects the rising cost of insurance both to the employer/provider and to the companies themselves. Obviously, the rising cost of health care is part of the problem. For example, costs for the average hospital stay in most East Coast states currently range from $500 to $1,500 per day. Obviously, myriad factors contribute to these costs; however, these factors are secondary to the average consumer, who believes these costs are merely more evidence to prove a conspiracy to exploit the health care customer/patient.

Government's role in health care will become even more prominent and have more effects on the health care business. Whenever an industry is perceived as being either unethical or unfair, government intervention is usually demanded to preserve the rights of the political constituency. A recent example of this phenomenon is a campaign by a New York City government official to stamp out (in his terms) "administration malpractice" of hospitals. This official is referring to hospitals in his borough that in his opinion raise costs unnecessarily, provide unacceptable levels of service to customer/patients, and overcharge them. Such an action could cause an interesting trend nationally if this official's plan is put into effect.

In another segment of the health care field, nursing homes have come under tremendous scrutiny in terms of their licensing procedures and operating practices. Many such facilities are currently barraged by large volumes of legislation and governmental compliance regulations. One administrator for a major midwestern facility recently told the author that more than two hours of every workday are spent on government compliance, whether in the form of report preparation, a meeting, or a series of phone calls. Such regulation and legislation might in fact be warranted; however, the administrator and facility perceived as unethical, suspected of dubious administration practices, or deemed less than aboveboard will be the object of even more scrutiny and face increasing demands to act ethically and morally.

Finally, the health care community itself has reacted en masse to the need for increased ethical standards and sound practices. Several governing bodies have set forth standards and programs that encourage ethical actions and the fair provision of services. These affect all facets of facility operations including marketing, care provision, human resources management, and financial administration. Furthermore, these institutions are providing education in various areas of ethical behavior and are encouraging professional organizations to implement a system of wide-ranging educational programs and informational packages on ethical standards as they relate to nonmedical activities.

The organization that takes health care ethics seriously and installs a comprehensive system of managerial ethics will survive and thrive in the 1990s. The organization that ignores ethical standards or uses standards that merely offer cosmetic appeasements to ethical demands will eventually suffer the consequences of being short-term smart but long-term foolish. Due to close scrutiny, industry regulation, and the demand of the health care business environment's principal player—the customer/patient—the ethically delinquent organization is doomed to fall by the wayside.

Ethics and the Premier Health Care Organization

In responding to consumer demand, the media, the government, and the health care community itself, the successful health care organization must embrace a strong organizationwide system of ethical management. Health care customer/patients, already skeptical of the health care business and the rapid change that has befallen local community providers over the past 15 years, are likely to be even more attuned to the ethical standards of providers. Particularly in situations in which consumers pay more of the cost for health care, expectations for high-quality care and optimum health care services will be even higher. Therefore, it is imperative that organizations embrace a strong set of ethics as part of their corporate culture and daily practices.

The health care business has always maintained a prominent tradition of strong ethical standards, from the Hippocratic oath to modern-day technology and the emergence of medical ethicists. However, much of this focus has been addressed to medical procedures and medical practices. As noted earlier, the need for an even broader perspective on ethics in all parts of the organization is required by today's marketplace. Furthermore, the business of health care, as its name implies, has as its main objective the provision of a service and a product that are unique in nature and humanistic in scope. From the standpoint of the consumer, it is easy to see where ethics must be applied in all marketing situations, in customer/patient relations, in service to the local community, and in the public's perception of health care. The organization perceived as being lax in ethical standards and moral conduct will surely suffer from the word-of-mouth publicity and media attention that such organizations merit. Furthermore, if the adjectives *inattentive, unconcerned,* or *insensitive* become commonplace in describing the local health care institution, a reputation will emerge that is contrary to the facility's business growth or a healthy bottom line.

In a similar vein, it is essential that the health care organization have ethical standards in its financial operations. An organization that overcharges patients or does not employ empathetic billing practices, for example, can surely be seen as unfair and interested in money only. This is again a negative perception that can quickly lead to loss of business in an extremely competitive marketplace. Moreover, the organization seen as having poor fiscal responsibility and inadequate financial controls can suffer from the perception that the organization has "money to burn" and is injudicious in the allocation of income it receives from its customer/patient community. In essence, this can be equated to abuse of the public trust and the community goodwill that support the health care organization.

Likewise, the institution's creditor and vendor relationships can be affected by poor financial control and lack of ethical standards. If vendors are not paid properly or dealt with justly, the hospital can earn a reputation as a "deadbeat" provider. Lack of attention to ethical behavior in this regard can certainly cause problems in terms of meeting supply needs, maintaining logistical support, and retaining purchasing relationships.

Another aspect of hospital operations that can be affected by questionable ethical practices is the purchasing operation, which is very visible and must adjudicate between an assortment of potential suppliers and vendors. Favoritism, whether real or imagined, can draw negative publicity for the hospital and, once again, stain the institution's reputation. Other parts of the operation—outpatient services, environmental services, dietary services, and the entire gamut of daily operations—can be affected in similar ways. The ethical standards and practices advocated in this book certainly apply to each and every phase of the operational part of a hospital or health care organization. Without question, lack of attention to any one of these areas can cause major problems for the entire organization, as later chapters of this book demonstrate.

An absence of a corporate culture that embraces a strong ethical foundation can be seen as detrimental to the health care organization as a whole, certainly to the most important component of the organization—its human resources. Most health care professionals are motivated not only by money and prestige, but also by the knowledge that they work for a strong ethical organization. In this regard, ethics are almost a lure for recruitment in that individuals will be attracted to work for an organization perceived as being "clean" from an ethical and moral standpoint. Most health care professionals are wise enough to realize that associating with an ethically questionable organization will be detrimental to their career progression and to their professional reputation. Furthermore, most of these well-motivated professionals are not eager to work in an organization whose individual employees do not share their ethical and moral convictions.

Lack of an ethical foundation within a medical facility can be the cause for high levels of employee turnover, because individuals may be asked to do things they perceive as being morally wrong or contrary to the true spirit of the health care profession. A health care organization with a strong training and development program in the ethics and standards of hospital services proves its commitment to ethics rather than merely paying lip service to the term or taking merely cosmetic measures.

In a recent project completed by the author's firm at a major Catholic hospital in Detroit, the author was asked to incorporate the hospital's organizationwide ethical standards into the performance evaluation scheme. As a result, the firm designed strong quantitative measures by which ethical practices were rewarded on the performance evaluation, in a fashion similar to measures for task accomplishment and goal achievement.

The use of quantitative measures for ethical behavior is more than a trend—it is a motivator for the "good people" in the organization and a method by which to motivate all employees toward strong ethical performance. The adage, "It's not what you do, it's how you do it," is never truer than in the case of ethical practices throughout a health care institution. The human resources of a good organization are motivated by ethical action; they strive to accomplish it in everyday activities and thus should be rewarded in concrete terms—at performance evaluation time and with a boost in their compensation level. Later chapters of this book demonstrate this particular dynamic in action and review a practical system for its implementation.

In many health care organizations, religious affiliation or a long-standing tradition of high-quality health care and selfless service is the basis for ethical standards of business. An institution that lacks such a system of management yet maintains a public stance of being an ethical provider risks being perceived as hypocritical and phony both in its intentions and in its execution of health care services. It is easy for an organization to mount a mission statement on a plaque for display in the admissions area or to include the statement in promotional literature, but it is more difficult to make ethical standards of conduct a reality throughout the organization.

All health care organizations indeed have a mandate to embrace strong ethical standards for their entire organization at both the individual and departmental levels. Executives and managers naturally set the pace, provide the role models, and enforce the standards, so it is their responsibility likewise to undertake a strong ethical system of management that can serve as an example for staff members and as a beacon for the customer/patients. Whereas such stated aims as "a sense of mission," "the winning edge," and "professionalism" ring prominently throughout the health care sector, the health care manager can quickly realize that attention to and execution of sound ethical practices can accomplish all of these aims.

☐ People Management Skills

Aside from the important component of organizational ethics—and the need for what is later described in this book as "value-driven management"—is the need for a more broad-based progressive management strategy that incorporates innovative people management. The health care manager must make certain that all of her or his assigned human resources are providing the health care organization with premium productivity and high-level performance in a long-term, mutually beneficial manner. This mutual benefit should extend to every level of the organization. That is to say, each employee should feel motivated by his or her manager as well as satisfied with the opportunities for skills development on the job; the manager should benefit from the synergistic effect of an entire group of inspired professionals working cohesively; and the organization should reap the benefits of all professional contributions.

The need for innovative people management is easily seen every day in the health care workplace as well as in professional journals and publications. Personnel shortages alone indicate the crying need for efficient staff motivation and management. In four seminars the author conducted for professional health care organizations within a two-week period in Canada, Ohio, New Jersey, and Texas, the question was posed to participating health care executives, "What personnel areas are currently understaffed due to human resources market supply in your organizations?" The answer in all four groups was the local colloquial equivalent of "You name it, we don't have it!"

Beyond addressing the challenge of recruitment, this book examines the manager's role in administering the organization's standards of employee development, compensation and performance evaluation, and basic personnel administration. The health care manager who is unarmed with new strategies in this area is doomed to professional failure, which can be manifested as employee apathy, uninspired performance, departmental productivity lapses, even high turnover rates. Compounded across the organization, this failure comprises a too-familiar formula for the demise of the nonprogressive health care organization.

Responsibility for creative and effective human resources management rests not with the personnel department of a health care organization but with every health care manager who supervises at least one employee. It is that manager's duty to provide a work environment that is fair, encourages maximum work contributions, and provides optimum opportunities for professional development.

Chapter 7 of this book provides a set of humanistic standards for innovative people management and further offers human resources strategies proven effective in progressive health care organizations. These standards and strategies are currently being employed successfully by managers across the organizational spectrum, from housekeeping to the executive suite. By understanding the pros and cons of these strategies and then exploring the programs and tactics used by health care leaders, the reader can formulate his or her sound perspective on human resources management and can use the practical tools for implementing individual progressive management strategies.

☐ Leadership Skills

The third component of progressive health care management is effective leadership skills, some facets of which generally include the following:

- A dynamic vision
- Stellar standards of business conduct
- Dedication to community and customer service
- A passion for high standards of quality
- Ability to take decisive action and to plan proactively

The basis for effective leadership is a set of value-based principles that meet the need for an ethical orientation throughout the health care workplace. One purpose of this book is to spell out these principles for the reader to incorporate into his or her own style of management.

Leadership, a subject of importance to both managers and executives, is specifically addressed at both the beginning and the end of this book, though its themes are woven throughout each chapter. Chapter 2 examines the 15 critical dimensions of leadership that serve as a framework for later discussions of value-driven management (chapter 3), employee motivational strategies (chapter 4), and other aspects of innovative people management (chapters 5–8). The concept of progressive leadership reappears in chapters 9 and 10 to explore community relations and business strategies from the executive point of view.

☐ Practical Applications

The need for progressive health care management strategies is on a par with the need for health care service quality. In fact, the two are interdependent, for without optimization of management skills, maximization of productivity and service is unattainable. This book assists readers to optimize their managerial strategies at the personal, departmental, and organizational levels and demonstrates a wide assortment of methods and tactics through explanation, practical examples, and case studies.

The systems described in this book enjoy the best validation of all— their proven effectiveness by leading health care organizations. This means that the time and financial investment spent on this book should provide a substantial return. The yield should include not only new ideas, but also strategies and tactics that are readily applicable in dealing effectively with some of the most complex challenges ever presented to executives and managers in the health care field.

Readers are encouraged to adapt and apply the information toward their specific situations. In general, readers should try to answer three basic questions as they read the text:

1. How does this information pertain to my role?
2. How can I use this information in my activities, as well as those of my staff?
3. What benefits can my organization/staff/department garner from pursuing one or more of these strategies?

☐ *Reference*

1. Arthur Andersen & Company. *Health Care in the 1990s.* Ann Arbor, MI: Health Administration Press, 1991, p. 3.

Chapter 2

The Organizational Leadership Imperative

As discussed in chapter 1, a progressive health care organization must have as its main proponent and guiding force a strong organizational leadership. It is incumbent upon leadership to provide a vision for the organization, set a specific mission, and provide key financial, human resources, and technical abilities so that the organization can meet its fundamental responsibility of providing stellar health care service to its constituency. Leadership in health care has been the premise for a number of journal articles, books, seminars, and professional development programs. Whereas these formats provide the health care executive and manager with a sound frame of reference relative to health care leadership, a realistic set of guidelines and practical strategies is needed to constructively develop leadership throughout the progressive health care organization.

This chapter first reviews the performance link between employees and the management and executive levels of the health care organization, and the combined effect of performance at each level on quality of care and customer/patient satisfaction. Later the chapter describes 15 critical dimensions of health care leadership that enhance management performance in any size facility and for any type of health care provider. In exploring specific applications, the chapter also presents the benefits and liabilities of implementing the 15 leadership dynamics and examines their importance to daily operations.

□ The Performance Link of Progressive Health Care Management

The most tangible way of comprehending the importance and interrelationship among employees, management, and leadership in a health care organization is to review what can be termed the *nuclear model of health care leadership,* demonstrated by figure 2-1. The all-encompassing entity in the model is the organization itself. The organization's executive leadership, its board of directors, and other guiding forces are all responsible for establishing the mission of the organization and reinforcing this mission and its importance to all members, primarily to management. In this connection, it is imperative that the facility's leadership group provide a set of corporate cultural norms and performance values (20 of which are defined in appendix A) that are recognizable, fully developed, and practically applicable to the conduct of work performance. In doing so, the organization provides for its employees a common vision and a sense of direction.

More specifically, the leadership should provide performance systems that allow each employee to realize his or her fullest potential as well as a system to reward performance. This provision includes performance

Figure 2-1.   The Nuclear Model of Health Care Leadership

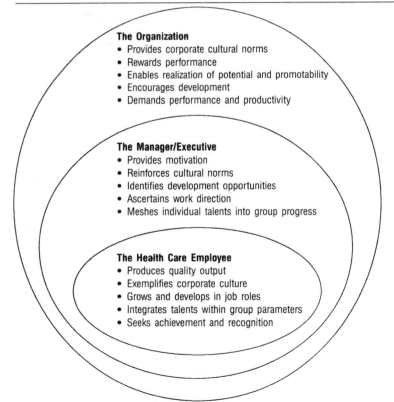

The Organization
- Provides corporate cultural norms
- Rewards performance
- Enables realization of potential and promotability
- Encourages development
- Demands performance and productivity

The Manager/Executive
- Provides motivation
- Reinforces cultural norms
- Identifies development opportunities
- Ascertains work direction
- Meshes individual talents into group progress

The Health Care Employee
- Produces quality output
- Exemplifies corporate culture
- Grows and develops in job roles
- Integrates talents within group parameters
- Seeks achievement and recognition

evaluation systems that not only measure attainment of elements of the job description but also encourage performance that is ethical (or value-driven) and comprehensive in scope. Such a system also rewards excellent performance during crises as well as for other significant contributions. Thus, the organization's standards should mandate high performance, measurable quality, and maximum productivity. As already noted, an important aspect of achieving these standards is the development of leadership skills.

Leadership that provides a clear vision, formulates a clear mission, and insists on high standards of quality and value- driven performance will achieve success within the health care business setting. A vision and a mission that are communicated clearly will encourage employees to perform at their maximum potential, achieve defined rewards, and embrace the organization as an important aspect of their lives. This in turn naturally provides strong motivation and inspiration to the employee for long-term success and long-term contributions to the organization.

The larger of the two inner spheres in figure 2-1 represents the manager/executive, whose differing roles are easily defined by exploring the attributes of their respective labels. That is to say, the title *manager* is derived from the Latin word *manus,* meaning "hand." The stellar health care manager is indeed a "hands-on" supervisor who is attuned to the needs and desires of his or her employees, understands the importance of the department's contribution, and knows intrinsically the keys to success for departmental achievement.

On the other hand, the executive is charged with executing action. Fundamentally, this entails studying plans and directives that link the employee to the "big picture" of the organizational imperative. The executive must work with the manager in meshing individual talents into the work and progress of the group, ascertaining departmental direction, identifying development opportunities for managers, reinforcing cultural norms, and providing motivation to all lines of report. Both the manager and the executive are basic administrators of the programs set forth by the upper echelons of organizational leadership.

At the center of the nuclear model in figure 2-1 is the employee. The role of every health care employee—who is unique to American industry in scope of technical expertise, dedication, work ethic, and commitment to mission—is to provide quality input to the management team on key work activities, along with quality output of work production. The individual should seek achievement and recognition throughout the work group retrospective to his or her talents and abilities and work contribution. Employees should also strive to integrate their talents within the group parameters and to ensure that their individual contribution is in sync with departmental and work group goals. Additionally, the stellar health care employee seeks to grow and develop in the job role by constantly enriching and enhancing his or her talents, job scope, and professional development.

Each employee is unique in that he or she represents the organization throughout the community. Health care itself is unique in that it is a public trust and is in a position of high visibility throughout the American collective psyche. Specifically, this means that in every community across the nation a citizen probably knows where a health care organization is located, may know people who work there, and may have a distinct opinion on how effective a local health care provider is. In this sense each health care employee is a public relations representative of an organization and, perhaps, the most visible link to the provider's customer/patient. With that in mind, it is imperative in a progressive health care organization that the individual employee serve as an example of excellence and embody the corporate cultural norms and performance values of the organization. After all, the decision to use a specific facility (a decision with an increasingly broad range of options) is often based on the interaction that a potential customer/patient has had with a member of that facility.

Some interesting parallels exist between the nuclear model of health care leadership in figure 2-1 and the nuclear model of atomic energy. For example, any turbulence that occurs outside an atom is reflected throughout the entire atomic structure. Likewise, the turbulence that affects a health care organization from the outside—the media, societal demands, and other external dynamics—has a profound effect on the entire structure of the organization, from employee to manager to executive to board of trustees. Furthermore, any internal changes in the atomic structure affect the entire atom, and any changes within a health care organization typically affect every member of the organization.

Similarities also exist between the various layers of an atomic structure and the layers of a health care organization. For example, if one layer of an atom is in conflict with another layer, destruction of the atomic structure takes place. A weak management, staff, or executive layer in a health care organization can also be destructive. The external turbulence alluded to above has even more specific implications, in that any upset of the outermost layer of an atomic structure can cause an explosion. In an equally dramatic fashion, an explosion can occur within an organization if outside forces act on the organization's outside layers—that is, the board of directors and the executive level—causing a harmful reaction (such as conflicting opinions or objectives). Finally, an implosion occurs in an atom when the nucleus reacts violently or splits. Any seasoned manager knows that conflict, lack of vision, low morale, or any of a multitude of problems among employees/staff can cause the implosion of a health care organization. Employee strife can mean loss of productivity, adverse union activity, high turnover, or an assortment of other ills that can plague the organization exponentially across all lines.

Without doubt the successful medical facility is marked by active employee participation, feedback, sound communication strategies, and a clear direction. From a general viewpoint, there is little argument that these are good objectives and credible ideals to which all health care organizations can aspire. However, specific strategies must be used to ensure that leadership is continuous, consistent, and constructive throughout all levels of the organization.

☐ Critical Dimensions of Health Care Leadership

Throughout this book, various strategies, systems, and practices are presented that can be adopted to enhance the performance of a progressive health care organization. A logical starting point is to consider a set of 15 critical dimensions of health care leadership:

1. Makes timely decisions
2. Can interact, inspire, and instruct
3. Understands and adheres to "bottom-line" requirements
4. Relates and is responsive to diverse personalities
5. Can anticipate and resolve problems proactively
6. Thrives on change and challenge
7. Manages conflict quickly and resolutely
8. Utilizes various and effective forms of motivation and inspiration
9. Can organize and present creative thought
10. Can get optimum performance from employees
11. Thrives on action; does not shun or seek the spotlight
12. Demands drive, desire, determination, and discipline of action
13. Makes the tough call and works through resistance and adversity
14. Sees the big picture; that is, the organizational relevance in *all* work activities
15. Demonstrates humanity with appropriate emotional responses, but is *always* creditable

The remainder of this chapter describes each dimension, discusses its requirements and importance, looks at its benefits, and—most important— examines how its misuse affects the manager and the health care business environment.

Making Timely Decisions

With the constant change in the health care management setting, and the complexity of issues that confront leaders daily in that setting, the ability to make correct decisions in a timely way is paramount. This includes the aptitude for collecting pertinent data quickly and effectively, weighing several options and viewpoints on the same issue, and assessing the best method to address a challenge. To bring this ability to the health care leadership role, credibility is garnered by the leader's staff, and the leader encourages staff commitment to the plan of action. Leaders who have this ability can take advantage of an array of business opportunities and have the latitude to pursue work activities proactively and progressively. Timeliness of decision making eliminates activity backlog, evidenced in a workplace where decisions are made slowly (if at all) and the work unit is constantly catching up to its responsibilities. Because health care organizations must do more with less, it is imperative that all leaders *truly* take charge of their areas of responsibilities in every situation.

Health care leaders who seesaw and procrastinate will have their competence and leadership abilities questioned by their staff. This results not only in loss of credibility but, in some cases, organizational mutiny as individuals make unauthorized decisions and other lapses occur in the chain-of-command process. Business opportunities might be missed, such as having the use of resources that might be available only in a certain time frame (the oft-cited "window of opportunity"), or accessing physical or financial resources that might not be available later. As a result, a business outcome might fall short of the potential results. Sometimes the positive effects of efficiency can be sabotaged when resources are overused or misspent in a plan of action that could have deferred to a more timely plan.

On an interpersonal level, the health care leader who fails to make timely decisions also risks negative assessment by peers. For example, other managers will avoid working closely with this type of leader out of fear that his or her judgment errors and mistimed actions will adversely affect their own endeavors. The overall effect of staff and peer mistrust on the work group is conflict, lack of direction, poor morale, and over-reliance on individual rather than group motivation, all of which will hamper productivity and performance and in turn jeopardize the entire organization.

Interacting with, Inspiring, and Instructing Employees

Again, the necessity to do more with less mandates that all human resources in a health care organization must be completely developed from a professional standpoint as well as from an overall health care business perspective. With this in mind, it is vital that all health care leaders demonstrate ability to interact with all employees, inspire top performance and continual professional growth, and instruct their charges on all technical and job-related activities. The latter includes not only current professional responsibilities but also instruction and orientation to changing dynamics in the health care business and how they affect an individual's job position. It also means addressing topics that might affect the individual as he or she progresses through the organization, by means of either promotion or expansion of duties. With training dollars limited by business realities and recognition that the best professional training takes place on the job, the main responsibility for employee education rests with the health care leader.

As demonstrated throughout this book, inspiration presents itself in many ways to the health care employee, mostly in the form of motivation. The principal responsibility for motivation of individual staff members lies with the health care leader, who ultimately must provide the impetus for group achievement and performance. Instruction on new techniques and various aspects of the health care setting are motivating factors in and of themselves, as is the underlying concern for employee growth demonstrated by on-the-job professional instruction. In most cases, the work group in which training and development is encouraged and facilitated by the leader is well motivated. It is also dependable, marked by consistency of performance, excellence of execution, and clearly defined professional productivity. An organization composed of several such units not only will survive in the difficult, sometimes uncharted, course of health care; it will also thrive and produce outstanding service to its customer/patient community.

The health care leader must strive to interact with all staff members in order to understand the particular developmental needs of each one and the most effective approach in enhancing that individual's development. With an ever-expanding spectrum of workers in the health care organization in regard to background and level of expertise, the leader must be able (at minimum) to relate to staff needs and (at maximum) to understand their professional and personal goals for achievement. The leader who has this knowledge and uses the workplace as a classroom, place of business, and forum for inspiration and personal satisfaction will ultimately provide the organization with outstanding departmental performance and overall excellence. Side benefits include an atmosphere that promotes knowledge as a value, thus encouraging all employees not only to learn but to instruct others. Consider, for example, the new employee who ultimately learns the ins and outs of a job from observing others in the same position. This basic principle is reinforced positively by a work group devoted to positive interaction and instruction, a group whose exemplar has been established by the most visible person in the organizational structure—the leader. This obviously also contributes to top performance across the board.

On the opposite side of the coin, health care work units deprived of effective interaction, inspiration, and instruction are besieged with problems. Without instruction, health care professionals do not grow to see their organizations, specifically as personified by their leader, as being interested in their growth and professional development. Poor performers are not given the opportunity to enhance their performance, mid- range performers will never be afforded the opportunity to raise their level of performance, and stellar employees will eventually leave the organization for one that will provide superior growth and development opportunity. As a totality, the work unit becomes stagnant and not only fails to grow but actually regresses due to lack of development in the face of increasing challenges.

Lack of interaction with staff, or too much negative interaction between the leader and employees, dampens positive motivation and inspiration for good performance. Lack of spirit among the entire work group can cause a health care professional eventually to leave the organization or deteriorate to routine poor performance. This trend will extend throughout the entire work group to stifle interdependence between work group members, which dissipates teamwork, cooperation, and loyalty among all staff members. Once again, absent positive action in the areas of interaction, inspiration, and instruction, progressive action in the workplace will suffer, choking off productivity and growth. Eventually, personnel turnover rates will rise, which will affect the organization in its entirety.

Understanding and Adhering to Bottom-Line Requirements

With fiscal resources becoming scarcer, health care executives and managers must understand the importance and basic responsibility of good fiscal management. Virtually everything a health care manager administers has a specific bottom-line relevance, even human resources. A poor hiring process, for example, can cost a manager countless dollars in recruitment costs, training costs, benefits enrollment, and downtime. A turnover situation is also costly. Wasted physical and fiscal resources can cost an organization countless dollars and reflect management incompetence.

A manager who understands the bottom-line requirements of his or her position knows the critical numbers that affect managerial performance and can set quantitative goals. Knowing that cost-effectiveness and fiscal efficiency are top priorities, such a manager uses allocated resources wisely by making strong projections, adhering to the budget, and protecting the organization's fiscal assets. By example, this individual demonstrates that waste, at all levels and across all financial lines, is to be avoided—without sacrifice to quality, however. In fact, quality output will be achieved through the intelligent use of fiscal resources. Managers who make good budget reports and fiscal projections understand the critical numbers relative to their sphere of influence in the organization.

To achieve optimal use of resources, a strong health care leader must be innovative—that is, work with the resources at hand (particularly the fiscal resources) rather than trying to be overly creative with resources not allocated or those allocated to another sector of the organization. In short, this individual can mix the mission with the means, that is, accomplish the mission and set goals with the fiscal allocations on hand without compromising quality.

On the negative side, an individual who goes overboard in terms of fiscal frugality at the expense of accomplishing a mission or specific objectives loses sight of intelligent fiscal management. A manager incapable of fiscal prudence places the entire organization and its resources at risk. Balancing between available fiscal resources and effective results is a difficult proposition for any health care manager. The manager who does not undertake this endeavor is not truly committed to the organization or to operational excellence.

Relating and Responding to Diverse Personalities

The health care workplace encompasses a wide assortment of personalities, from both a psychological and a sociological perspective. Health care can involve every demographic category, and actors can appear in the health care equation as either a customer/patient or an employee. Health care managers are charged with ensuring that all customer/patients receive high-quality care, including the area of interpersonal relations and measurable outcome, regardless of personality or sociological background. Likewise, all health care employees are entitled to the same opportunities for promotion and development without regard for personal or demographic variables.

Unfortunately, some health care employees tend to label not only diseases but personality types. Often this labeling is unfair because of the fast pace and inordinate pressure in the health care environment. To illustrate, figure 2-2 shows factions within a health care organization as labeled and categorized by the majority of organizational members. In this organization, a regressive atmosphere is apparent; animosity is the order of the day; and avoidance and conflict overshadow cooperation, communication, and quality of care.

An exemplary leader will avoid labels and instead objectively assess the tendencies and proclivities of the individuals he or she is dealing with, be it a patient or an employee. This leader will possess listening skills and perceptual ability, which will allow him or her to deal with a variety of personality types and a wide spectrum of cultural differences among the workplace populace. Such people skills help motivate and facilitate communication among members of the work unit or staff.

Figure 2-2. Perceptual Profile of the Regressive Health Care Organization

CEO/Administration

- No vision
- Egocentric
- Indecisive/lacks strength
- Lacks sensitivity/empathy

Finance/ Accounting	Physicians/ Nursing	Human Resources	Technical Support	Marketing/ Operations

• $-only mentality
• Insensitive
• Overly negative
• Closed-minded
	• Militant/elitist
	• Victims/martyrs
	• Nonparticipative
	• Combative/
	  contrary
		• Paper pushers
		• Unimaginative
		• No perspective
		• Process-oriented
			• Isolationists
			• Limited scope
			• No business
			  sense
			• No team spirit
				• Trend followers
				• Ill-defined
				  mission
				• Unrealistic
				• Flighty/frivolous

Attainment of the basic health care mission is the most important aspect of the daily life of any health care unit. That mission is to provide top-quality health care to any needy individual at any given time in any given situation. Therefore, the health care leader at any level must be perceived as being fair, equitable, and understanding in dealings with staff and in all interpersonal contact. Otherwise the leader risks being labeled as bigoted, ignorant, or insensitive. This perception can create a faction of discontent within the organization and in turn earn the department the unfortunate distinction of one (or more) of the labels shown in figure 2-2. Furthermore, the leader of this department will hire and promote individuals who have the same tendencies that he or she has. In the long run, this "halo effect" will produce a department of people who think alike, act alike, and are indifferent to outsiders and differing norms or personalities. The most prominent negative effect of this phenomenon is isolation from the total health care organization and disharmony with organizational objectives, values, or ideals.

Anticipating and Resolving Problems Proactively

An overused idiom of American business parlance is Murphy's law—in essence, anything that can go wrong will go wrong. As trite as this expression has become, it still holds profound significance for the health care leader on those days when it seems as though nothing goes right or according to plan. Therefore, it is imperative that health care managers have a proven ability to anticipate problems and resolve them quickly and efficiently.

A manager truly in tune with the department's objectives can foresee difficulties that might sidetrack the work group and work situation and plan an attack to address the problems—including preparations for a plan B and a plan C if needed. Managers can enlist staff help in finding a solution so that the problem does not become an ongoing issue throughout the work group and a thwart to future success. Chapter 6 discusses particular strategies that can be used by the leader in this regard and provides further criteria that establish proactive problem solving as part of the daily regimen.

Conversely, the manager who cannot anticipate problems and respond proactively in their resolution is destined to rely on reactionary strategies. That is, the circumstances will present themselves, the negative situations will take hold, and the manager is in a position of simply trying to survive rather than thriving. Such an individual will be perceived as a weak or incompetent leader. Consequently, confidence in the leader and faith in his or her ability will be diminished throughout the organization, most notably among the staff. In the long term, the credibility of this proverbial "weak link" will be questioned throughout the entire organization.

Thriving on Change and Challenge

Change, which is a feature of the health care environment, is both a motivator and a de-motivator. When it becomes overwhelming, or unreasonable, change can become a de-motivator. Effective management of change, including the way in which it is presented and addressed throughout the work group, is an important managerial asset. Chapter 5 discusses change and provides detailed strategies on how to manage its presence within the health care organization.

Challenge, in the form of increased responsibility and demand for action, is another prominent factor in the health care workplace. In order for organizations to do more with less, it is imperative that managers embrace a maximum level of challenge. This is important not only from an organizational perspective, where the individual takes on as much responsibility as possible; it is also important for the individual's leadership development because challenge provides the foremost opportunity to grow and learn within the scope of the job. Health care leaders who thrive on challenge welcome it, manage its aspects, and learn significantly from the experience. In turn, they challenge their employees, motivate them toward a success, and act as a facilitator in the educational opportunity that challenge presents.

Managers who avoid challenge are doomed to mediocrity in the health care business setting. Given that challenge is a factor in the everyday life of a health care organization, an appropriate analogy can be made between it and fire. If fire—a basic element—is used correctly it can provide heat or cooking fuel, among a variety of positive applications. Used inappropriately, fire can be destructive.

With that in mind, if a manager is unable to harness challenge (a basic element) within a health care workplace, chances are that he or she is failing to motivate employees—or himself or herself—with proper job objectives that stretch abilities and optimize personal development. In effect, neither the manager nor the staff is providing the organization with the full range of possible contributions. In the short run this deficit will hurt productivity; in the long run it will severely cripple overall organizational development.

Managing Conflict Quickly and Resolutely

Conflict within a health care workplace must be managed quickly, fairly, and resolutely. Inability to do this causes the manager to be perceived as ineffective and unconcerned with the daily activities of the department. If conflict is allowed to fester, it can become a source of contention among workers. (Chapter 5 discusses conflict resolution in detail.) However, it is important to understand the elementary importance of conflict to leadership, and to recognize that the apathetic health care manager who does not manage conflict effectively risks animosity throughout the workplace and ineffective action from subordinates. Furthermore, both customer/patients and other members of the organization can clearly recognize conflict and its negative effects on performance.

The health care manager who can manage conflict effectively is seen as a take-charge individual and can often gain the confidence of staff and superiors. As an elementary part of human nature, conflict is bound to exist at all levels of the health care organization. It has numerous roots, various symptoms, and a wide variety of risks. A health care manager who handles conflict successfully and brings about a positive conclusion enhances his or her credibility, effectiveness of leadership style, management abilities, and overall staff productivity.

Utilizing Effective Forms of Motivation and Inspiration

Motivation and inspiration, as applied to the health care business setting, is a double-edged sword. On the positive side of the blade is the fact that most health care workers are motivated by an intrinsic desire to help their fellow human beings and provide stellar health care service. On the negative side is the fact that health care has become such an appealing target to the media and the public consciousness. One need only review the dynamics described in chapter 1 or follow the daily news media to see the negative manner in which health care is sometimes portrayed.

This negative press of course affects the average health care employee as well as the leader. With limited money to reward performance from the perspective of compensation and benefits, it is most important for the health care manager to implement reward systems that provide various forms of inspiration for staff performance and motivation for quality output. Throughout this book, specific motivational strategies and applications are detailed for the immediate use of managers and executives. This section explores the importance of motivation to the health care leader.

Foremost, the health care leader must be able to motivate a large group of people. This means that not only must group motivational and inspirational strategies be in place, such as providing a clear vision and suffusing a winning spirit throughout the work group, but strategies for individual motivation must be used as well. For example, a manager who tries to motivate 10 different people in 10 different ways is more apt to be successful than the manager who tries to motivate 10 different people in the same way. That is to say, each health care employee brings a particular set of objectives and desires to the workplace. Although there are some similarities, such as the need for a progressive workplace and fair compensation, these vary in terms of application and importance to the individual. Furthermore, each employee has a unique set of specific motivational keys that need to be pressed effectively by the manager. A manager who tries to use a blanket approach to motivation will run the risk of being perceived as phony, predictable, or insensitive to the needs of individual staff members.

In an arena where resources are limited, motivation is a key to productivity and quality. It then becomes incumbent on a manager to come up with specific strategies and approaches that will inspire greater employee performance. As the health care business comes under more and more scrutiny from a variety of external sources, it will become even more important for health care leaders to learn motivational strategies for attaining maximum productivity, optimum quality, and top employee performance in the workplace.

Organizing and Presenting Creative Thought

The health care setting that requires managers and leaders to do more with less has an inherent mandate for leadership that can organize and present creative thought. For example, creative thought is necessary to solve problems — an individual who lacks creativity cannot offer creative solutions. Conversely, an individual who is overly creative may be incapable of communicating so that others can understand and help resolve a dilemma. An individual who is "too creative" is seen as being "all over the place" and not a usable resource throughout the health care organization.

An innovative thinker is a wellspring of new ideas. Others in the organization will be inspired to use this person as a checkpoint or sounding

147, 75 8

board for their new ideas and as a source of inspiration to find better ways of accomplishing the mission. This process promotes organizational growth and development, prompts the leader's peers to grow within their own areas of responsibility, and of course encourages the staff to be imaginative yet pragmatic in their outlook and perception of job responsibilities.

In a business where change and increasing demands are routine, an individual who neither thinks creatively nor encourages others to do so not only is a liability to the organization but a liability to himself or herself.

Getting Optimum Performance from Employees

Chapter 6 will discuss the specifics of how to plan, prioritize, orient, and effect optimum performance through a systematic planning strategy. For now, it is important to recognize the value of these strategies to the leadership role.

An individual who can plan and prioritize staff actions, orient the staff, and effect desired performance increases his or her ability to analyze situations and arrive at the optimum way to achieve results. This individual applies his or her creative talents to set specific parameters for performance—that is, a list of tasks to be accomplished and a plan for expediting them.

Inability to plan, prioritize, orient staff, and effect desired performance can spell disaster for the leader. Others will be reluctant to follow someone who has no clear direction or fails to produce excellent results routinely. This in turn creates a norm where people will not be inspired to achieve top performance and will not seek to provide the organization with maximum return on investment and return for compensation dollars. Furthermore, department heads who cannot embrace this critical dimension of leadership cannot be counted on to contribute their department's best work to the overall organizational picture. As a result, a fracture forms in the organization because a piece of the organizational pie is either missing or defective. Not only do productivity and quality suffer, but the department is also labeled ineffective, unreliable, and inconsistent in its performance.

Referring back to the nuclear model (figure 2-1), it is vital that an organization have an overall strategic plan that delineates the responsibilities of each section of the organization and identifies a specific course of action and specific outcomes for the enhancement of management skills. This helps ensure that operational objectives are being achieved and, as will be shown later in this text, that the human resource development and performance aspects of plan achievement are also realized.

Thriving on Action

A stellar health care leader thrives on both the pressure and pace that are unique to the health care environment. With the increased demands and accelerating pace intrinsic to the health care business setting, leaders should be able to respond positively as the pace of action quickens and pressure increases. The health care business is very much in the public spotlight, from both a national and a local perspective. A health care manager is always visible to staff members and, more times than not, to the customer/patient. Even if a manager is not visible to the customer/patient, his or her work and departmental output usually are, either directly or indirectly.

An individual who shuns this high-profile action and its accompanying responsibility is destined for burnout, limitations on career advancement, or removal from the health care business sector. Managerial timidity sets a harmful precedent and sends a negative message to staff members — especially if the leader's response to crisis management is negligence and negative consequences.

Another angle of the "action scenario" is the leader who, constantly seeking the spotlight, is perceived as egocentric and self-serving in a profession that prides itself on selflessness. A stellar health care leader understands that the basic objective is to enable and empower employees to achieve an optimum level of performance, which in turn will benefit the customer/patient to the maximum potential. There is little room in this equation for self-serving egotism or self-aggrandizement, and one who follows this course is destined to take a big fall.

Demanding Drive, Desire, Determination, and Discipline

The performance value of industry and the work ethic are two factors that are integral to the success of any health care organization or department. It is the responsibility of the leader to ensure that these factors are part of the department's norm and a standard throughout the health care workplace. Customer/patients can perceive whether maximum effort is given on behalf of their physical well-being by looking first at the caliber of effort given by the health care staff as evidenced by output and effect.

The executive or manager should seek to instill a basic drive in his or her staff so that each worker demonstrates a high degree of self-initiative and independent motivation toward accomplishing all set tasks and objectives. The positive effect of this drive will spread throughout the organization. However, a health care leader who demands drive and self-initiative from staff but fails to set an example through his or her own diligence is easily pegged as a hypocrite or a phony.

A leader should desire to achieve the best possible results in any given situation. This desire is earmarked by a hunger to develop appropriate professional expertise and technological know-how so as to provide the customer/patient with optimum health care. Again, the extent to which this work ethic is in place will be reflected positively or negatively, depending strictly on the example set forth by the leader.

Determination is defined in this context as the overt intention to succeed despite situational obstacles. Determination, evidenced by a strong commitment on the part of the leader and his or her staff, is readily identified by a customer/patient or by another department or colleague. Individuals seen as being determined are usually seen as being dedicated and therefore consistent and dependable. Obviously, lack of determination, earmarked by overt willingness to forgo working persistently through obstacles can earn a reputation for weak leadership skills.

Leaders who instill drive, desire, and determination in the work ethic—without becoming zealots—enforce a strict set of standards that benefit not only customer/patient service delivery, but also employee development. Discipline equates to efficiency on the job and proper optimization of resources, both of which drive desirable performance values in a progressive health care organization. As turbulent times continue to affect the health care work setting, these leadership qualities are not only desirable but essential to success.

Making the Tough Call

In the health care setting, leaders are asked daily to make decisions that might prove to be unpopular or complex in scope, or that might have potentially negative effects. Managers who put the organizational imperative at the forefront of their responsibilities demonstrate a sense of integrity to the organization and its goals. An easier way to illustrate this point is to look at the liabilities incurred by a leader who refrains from making the tough call.

Leaders who do not like to make a tough call run the risk of losing credibility throughout the organization because they do not meet challenges head-on or expend extra effort. Furthermore, they may be seen as lacking a firm position and having no courage of convictions. In the long run, they will not be relied on for tough action, and inevitably will be excluded from crisis situations or management dilemmas. In such a case, the organization *and* the manager lose.

On the other hand, the manager who makes the tough call and works at achieving goals in the face of adversity gains the trust of staff as well as peers. Furthermore, upper management and the higher echelons of the organization will recognize this leader as a "go-to" person— someone to go to when organizational interests need to be at the forefront. Such a leader will naturally gain support and be seen as reliable and consistent in crisis situations.

Due to increased scrutiny and a changing regulatory environment, health care management is more intricate than ever. Managers who can make the tough call without worrying about their popularity and work through resistance and adversity will be valued commodities to their organizations.

Seeing the Big Picture

Oftentimes in health care, the activities of an individual department are not seen as being integral to the entire organization. This perception can cause disparate feelings between the work group and the rest of the organization. Moreover, it is a lost opportunity for motivation in that an employee's knowledge of how his or her efforts affect the entire organization's ability to provide services is a strong motivator at any level or in any job in a health care organization. Remember, health care professionals are driven primarily by their desire to help those in need of health care services. With that in mind, attaching relevance to the big picture fuels this motivating factor.

It is sometimes difficult for individuals to understand how their job role affects the entire scope of organizational operation. Therefore, leaders must look for opportunities to illustrate to employees how the big picture is supported by individual efforts. This can be done through anecdote or by any other strategies delineated later on in this book.

Relating individual activities to the big picture also reinforces standards of quality throughout the work group and the organization. In essence, if a health care employee understands why his or her job is so important, the odds are that that employee will take every opportunity to be effective in supporting the organization's mission.

Demonstrating Humanity

A final critical dimension in health care leadership is the manager's ability to show that he or she is indeed human. Giving appropriate emotional support serves as a motivator and shows that the organization is run by people, not machines. Good leadership accomplishes this by exhibiting neither overbearing nor "bleeding heart" emotionalism, that is, by understanding that every situation cannot be treated as a crisis or life-or-death event. Appropriate emotions include encouragement, elation, and enthusiasm. Certainly, negative emotions such as disappointment and dissatisfaction also may be appropriate, depending on the specific situation.

An individual devoid of emotion will not be held in esteem because appearing robotlike is a distinct liability in a people-intensive business such as health care.

☐ Practical Applications

Progressive leadership is integral to the success of any health care organization. By studying the basic concepts of leadership and planning specific strategies, as this book continues to do in succeeding chapters, the health care manager or executive can ensure that an effective and forward-looking leadership style prevails.

The following list of practical applications may be used as a starting point for examining the extent to which the critical dimensions of health care leadership are present in your organization or department:

1. Review the material in this chapter and assess yourself, your reporting supervisors, if any, and your organizational leadership.
2. Refer to other chapters in this book for guidance on specific application of these 15 dimensions of leadership.
3. Utilize these dimensions as part of your selection strategy for new supervisors, both from candidates already in your organization and candidates from the external health care job marketplace.
4. Incorporate these dimensions of leadership into your performance appraisal scheme.
5. Use the list of 15 leadership dimensions as a basis for discussion with your peers or subordinate leaders.
6. Incorporate these 15 dimensions in all leadership training and leadership assessment activities.
7. Periodically review this information with respect to your own leadership activities and those of your subordinate leaders.
8. Study the 20 organizational performance values in chapter 3 and appendix A of this book and also define your own leadership criteria based on the 15 dimensions.
9. Prioritize which of these dimensions should be key strengths in particular situations. For example, which 5 of these 15 dimensions would be most important in a personnel manager? Which 5 would be least important in a nursing director? Would all 15 be important in both positions?
10. As appropriate, elicit employee suggestions about these leadership dimensions. Which ones are the most inspirational and/or important to them? Which ones do they perceive as being important from an organizational point of view? In a similar vein, executives can assess how board members feel about these dimensions and can perhaps garner their input as well.

☐ Chapter 3

Value-Driven Management

Rising customer/patient demand for optimum health care delivery, as well as increased employee expectations of the parent organization, has created wide-scale interest in values and ethics in health care management. Health care intrinsically has a moral commitment to society; in fact, medical ethics dates back to ancient societies. The issue of *value-driven management*—a system of administration and daily management practices that embody personal values, humanistic standards, business norms, and executive principles—is extremely important not only from an ethical viewpoint but from a purely business perspective as well.

This chapter explores a set of 20 performance values that can be applied in hiring, directing, developing, and evaluating health care professionals at all levels of the organization. (These 20 values are the subject of appendix A.) Four categories are reviewed:

1. *Personal values* are ethical standards an individual brings to the job based on his or her upbringing, education, and experience.
2. *Humanistic standards* are guidelines for understanding, accepting, and relating to other people.
3. *Business norms* are standards of conduct for fair business practices on the part of the organization.
4. *Executive principles* cover the ethical standards for leadership strategies and conduct.

The information in this chapter, along with the definition of terms and the worksheets in appendix A, enable the health care manager to implement and reinforce critical standards to promote a successful organization.

☐ Personal Values

Personal values include decency, fortitude, industry, integrity, and knowledge.

Decency

Health care professionals whose personal actions reflect a basic sense of right and wrong as it relates to their professional responsibilities are daily reminders of the value of decency in the workplace. Through their treatment of other people—whether a housekeeper, a CEO, or a customer/patient—they demonstrate a high regard for others as human beings and health care organization players. Implicit in this sentiment is the perception that everyone in the organization is vital to the success of the institution. Professionals with a sense of decency show no favoritism and constantly seek to apply their talents to the quest of helping those who need premium health care services.

Tact is another indicator of decency. For example, when describing people the diplomatic leader will refrain from using demeaning language or being overbearing. Even when faced with a delicate situation or a distasteful individual, the poised leader will use quick dispatch. In short, decency will prevail.

Decent leaders understand that money is not the most important factor in the health care business equation, that high-quality care is the top priority. Also, recognizing that human interaction is the most important exchange in a health care organization, they will act to provide a high standard of health care service and take any extra steps required to ensure maximum human interaction. In no instance will they let money requirements or time restrictions affect the quality of either of these important dimensions.

Decency is the foundation for a system of ethics in a progressive health care organization. Its absence is incongruous with the health care mission, and executives and managers at all levels should harness it for their team-building efforts within the organization.

Fortitude

The value of fortitude is demonstrated by an individual who brings a sound unpretentious quality of courage to the everyday workplace that enables the capacity to make tough decisions and seek the most ethical solution to any business challenge. This individual is patient in obtaining solid results and steadfast in constructing ethically optimum plans. This value relates primarily to executives and managers but must be embraced by any worker in the health care organization. The reason this value is important to all health care professionals is that many times, due to personnel shortages and the nature of the health care profession, individual workers at all levels are called on to make autonomous decisions. Therefore, they must have courage to make the call that is in the interest of good performance and sound ethical action. The positive

actions that arise from the sound use and practical application of fortitude are easy to discern in the health care manager.

A leader who possesses fortitude has the courage to examine every
conceivable angle of an issue before making a decision that could
adversely affect an employee. A variety of solutions must be examined
so as to come up with the best possible resolution rather than making
a snap judgment that might interfere with employee motivation.

A courageous leader is armed with self-knowledge, self-confidence,
and self-actualization. In short, this person is comfortable making decisions and taking action in the highest ethical traditions of health care
management; he or she also has a work history that indicates a propensity for making correct decisions in a number of situations. Furthermore,
he or she is not easily swayed by opposing personalities or dubious arguments. Staff and peers see in this leader a willingness to seek the most
progressive and ethical action to achieve optimum performance.

Industry

One whose work ethic demonstrates the value of industry serves as an
example for all members of the organization. He or she is singled out
by supervisors and executives as being an effective and efficient worker.
Effectiveness in the context of industry relates to productivity and quality of performance. *Efficiency* relates to the quantity of time and money
used in attaining set goals. An individual who has an ethical commitment to the value of industry does not waste resources, uses all resources
at hand, and shows the best possible production results.

Industrious employees consistently work at top level on all projects,
not just those of particular interest or benefit to them. They diligently
pursue all performance objectives, not just those that will enhance their
promotability or visibility within the organization. Such individuals make
the most of all opportunities, from attending weekly meetings and completing routine "administrivia" and paperwork to handling the most
pressing emergency situations and high-visibility opportunities for action.

In a similar fashion, diligent leaders never accept less than the best
results from subordinates. They challenge others as well as themselves
to always seek the higher ground with respect to efforts and results; this
practice relates to the managerial concept of progressive development.
The individual who truly has an ethical commitment to industry always
seeks to build progressively on his or her previous result. Even if that
prior outcome was fully acceptable and beneficial to the organization,
the industrious employee will always seek to top it. For example, an X-
ray technician who can perform a radiologic procedure efficiently and
effectively 10 times within a given period will aspire to 11 times as the
next standard of excellence. Persons with a high degree of industry are

constantly challenging themselves to gain better results and to create more efficient means of doing so.

From a purely ethical standpoint, this individual understands that half-stepping at any point along the chain of command cheats the organization and, ultimately, the customer/patient. He or she realizes that the health care business setting is no place for laziness, apathy, or a tendency to place politics above outcome. Due to the nature of the health care business in the 1990s and due to acute personnel shortages, without a high degree of industry among managers, staff, and hourly workers, a health care organization will take the quickest route to failure.

Integrity

Integrity is essential to the character of the health care manager, the hourly worker, and the entire organization. Unless it permeates every aspect of the organization, the organization's credibility will be questioned and its presence in the community will come under question.

A health care professional who utilizes integrity as part of everyday work strategy always presents accurate and documentable facts and figures as part of the rationale for objective decision making. These individuals refuse to accept unsubstantiated opinions or viewpoints and try to ascertain objectively the outcomes and establish consequences of any action taken.

In relationship to their supervisory responsibilities, they demand no less from their subordinates. If a subordinate wants supervisory approval on a proposed action, the honest health care manager will challenge the soundness of the course of action. This leader will encourage investigation and factual evidence over conjecture or subjective opinion.

The health care professional who maintains a high degree of integrity is honorable and candid in all business dealings and is willing to take an unpopular stand or make a tough decision. Honest managers share information and have no fear of presenting facts directly in any given situation. They exercise tact and compassion when delivering information or viewpoints of a sensitive nature. Furthermore, they can be relied on to tell the whole story, not just the acceptable or popular segments. In short, these individuals have an unfailing sense of honor that forbids them from lying, cheating the organization, or compromising a valued trust.

Knowledge

The final personal value is knowledge. A knowledgeable health care manager constantly pursues growth and development activities that strengthen business and technical acumen and personal enhancement. This individual realizes that there is something new to be learned every day and in every situation and that attaining as much knowledge as possible is a responsibility and a requirement of ethical leadership. There is an old Italian proverb that, loosely translated, states: "The walls that an individual puts up to keep others out are the same walls that keep that person in." This adage underscores the need for two- way communication in the attainment of knowledge.

Several practical actions are taken by the well-motivated health care manager or executive who embraces the value of knowledge. In general, this individual will take advantage of as many developmental activities as possible, from seminars to enlightening discussions. He or she will read as much as possible on significant issues and constantly seek opportunities to learn new methods, procedures, programs, and any other developments that might further the provision of premium health care services. Managers recognize the learning value in talking to an hourly employee or a customer/patient in the interest of gaining a perspective on how to better utilize a service or economize its efficiency. These conversations also reveal the needs and desires of customer/patients, their expectations, and their priorities in terms of the services and products they receive.

Knowledge-seeking health care managers always ask the right questions in business situations. They utilize open-ended questions in order to learn the rationale behind decisions made or actions taken. They do this to gain insight pertinent to their management responsibility and the delivery of health care and also to discover the depth of a particular situation or a course of action, a set of job responsibilities, or a specific health care program. By seeking to understand rationales and philosophies as well as objective facts, managers gain a wide perspective of knowledge in health care as well as increase their frame of reference for health care organizations' operations and procedures. This breadth of knowledge ultimately works to the benefit of the entire organization.

☐ Humanistic Standards

Humanistic standards include allegiance, compassion, dignity, introspection, and spirit.

Allegiance

In the health care setting, allegiance is the exercise of fidelity, through words and actions, to helping those in need and supporting those engaged in the provision of superior health care. An individual who embraces this principle is loyal to others in the workplace and is always willing to assist those who need assistance in the conduct of their professional duties. He or she gives maximum effort in individual and group activities that benefit the organization, seeing their work role as being intrinsic to the accomplishment of the organizational mission.

A person who has exemplified the characteristic of allegiance in the workplace is looked on by others in the organization as being someone who can be relied on in tough situations, depended on for advice or professional guidance, and entrusted with confidential or sensitive matters.

Another attribute of an individual who demonstrates allegiance in the workplace is willingness to act as a mentor to inexperienced personnel. For example, a number of health care workers have learned a great deal from technical training and schoolwork but have not had the opportunity to apply that knowledge in the workplace. To fill in the gap between theory and practical experience, a person more experienced and seasoned in the health care organization can act as a mentor. This is where ethical quality of allegiance is demonstrated by the individual who serves in the mentor capacity willingly and consistently. He or she sees this opportunity as another way of being committed to the organization and understands that from a business venue this will help the organization and the worker.

Compassion

Among all spheres of human endeavor, the health care field is truly a "people business." Without compassion on the part of executives and managers, employees may feel that their managers and administration do not care about them. Furthermore, work environments in which compassion is not a byword often suffer high turnover because the workplace is simply not a pleasant place to spend 8–10 hours each and every day.

Lack of compassion among coworkers and superiors also can be detected by the customer/patient. If a customer/patient perceives that the workers do not care for one another, they surely will conclude that the organization and its members do not care about them.

Individuals who display a high degree of compassion always listen to explanations and weigh decisions carefully when confronted with a people-intensive situation. They examine the perceptions and frame of reference of all of the players in a scenario and try to arrive at a fair decision. A compassionate individual will not apply the techniques of a "one-minute manager" but will appreciate the consequences of his or her decisions. He or she will also understand that nothing is more threatening to organizational morale than the perception that a person has been treated unfairly.

Compassion allows for ease of conversation with all coworkers and patients, regardless of cultural background or other frame of reference.

Compassionate people are sensitive in their dealings and can accept a variety of perceptions and viewpoints. However, they do not let compassion become a weakness in their management style; nor do they allow their good intentions to be exploited—for example, relaxing productivity or quality expectations.

Managers who lack compassion talk a good game about sensitivity, fairness, and the importance of people, but they fail to back up claims through example. For example, such managers rarely make time to discuss problems with those in need of help. Or they may inhibit freedom of expression among workers. In effect, they see people problems as a nuisance and have failed consistently to understand that people problems are often the number-one cause of management breakdown. An individual who lacks compassion will gravitate toward others who have a similar background.

Dignity

Managers with a proper degree of dignity give due respect to all members of the organization, from housekeepers to board members. They respect executives because of their responsibility for making critical decisions and devising plans that affect the overall organization. They also respect the individual employee who works hard every day to turn those plans into reality.

At the executive level, health care leaders must make certain that all reporting managers are acutely aware of the need to respect the dignity of individual employees. The same value must take hold at the managerial and supervisory levels. In turn, managers must be certain that employees understand that all coworkers are to be respected, assisted in times of need, and recognized for their importance to the organization. Managers can show their respect for employee dignity in a variety of ways. The most obvious way is to constantly seek opportunities to develop employees to their fullest professional and interpersonal potential.

The executive or manager in a health care setting must solicit information from a variety of sources on maintaining and increasing the "dignity quotient" throughout the organization. The primary source might be the employees themselves. By implementing employee surveys, group conversations, and individual discussions, the manager can get a firm charting on how the employees feel they are being treated. Topics might include employee attitudes, promotion opportunities on the job, and employee assessment of how well they are respected and appreciated by the organization. Another means might be to discuss with peers at other organizations how their employee relations are managed; that is, what methods other organizations use to help employees feel valued. A third method, quite simple in concept but unfortunately ignored widely by health care organizations, is executive retreats and management conferences at which managers address how they embrace the value of employee dignity and what lessons they have learned.

The discerning manager understands and reinforces through action the importance of individual dignity to the overall success and cohesiveness of the health care organization.

The manager who fails to appreciate the import of dignity throughout the workplace might demonstrate bias in giving respect to individuals. For example, he or she might show respect only for those who play a certain role or have a high degree of visibility in the organization. Ignoring the viewpoints of others, failing to appreciate their beliefs, being self-centered and self-aggrandizing—these are all actions that alienate employees and peers alike. Dignity, therefore, is important in helping to build a value-driven workplace and in fostering positive employee relations.

Introspection

An introspective individual constantly challenges himself or herself to attain the highest degree of professional achievement and maintain the best ethical standards in all situations. This individual is consistent in thinking through important issues, balancing consequences with actions, and tempering force with humanistic considerations. In short, health care managers who incorporate introspection into their daily strategy have a great degree of insight into their own actions and how those actions affect the work lives of subordinates, peers, and superiors. An introspective individual thinks before acting, weighs perceptions against facts, and puts the feelings and well-being of others at the top of the priority list.

In the tradition of Solomon, introspective individuals work systematically from general to specific dimensions before arriving at a just decision. Not only does this engender the respect of those individuals affected by the outcome of the decision, but the rationale developed for making the decision lends credibility to the final outcome. Also, respect is implicit for all individuals involved in the decision because, by virtue of the time taken to come to a decision, a manager has already indicated the importance of the decision's effect on those involved.

Introspective individuals are their own toughest critics. As already noted, they set high standards for themselves in terms of their performance and ethical conduct on the job. Without obsessing on the past, they seek to learn from the consequences of their actions, and they progressively develop a strong strategy for the ethical management of others. These individuals will have the courage (or fortitude) to objectively assess their performance and approach to their management duties. They constantly look for clues on how to better themselves as managers and people and respond to objective, well-meaning criticism and opinions on their management style.

Spirit

Spirited health care professionals usually maintain a steady upbeat attitude as appropriate. They come to work "charged up" for a full day's activities and leave personal problems at the door. They try to speak in positive terms as much as possible; whenever negative consequences or actions must be faced, they seem to turn them into a positive solution when possible. An agreeable sense of humor is usually on call to cheer up others when the need presents itself. All in all, they serve as a source of positive motivation and encouragement for others, they ignore "doom and gloom" projections, and rally to address a situation aggressively and optimistically. Their motto is "Quitters never win and winners never quit." With this in mind, they make several attempts to get a difficult job done, provided they believe the job is vital and ethically sound in nature. A spirited leader takes pride in the accomplishments of staff and peers and is happy for others' success and its effect on the organization. Finally, this individual will do everything possible in his or her sphere of responsibility to help encourage and further others' progress.

☐ Business Norms

Business norms include customer/patient commitment, forthright tactics, professional liberty, quality, and social awareness.

Customer/Patient Commitment

The successful organization, whether it is health care or another field, understands implicitly that the customer is at the top of the organizational chart. Without customers, no products and services are sold, no profits are generated, and businesses fold. Therefore, the first of the health care value-based business norms revolves around the customer/patient. This consumer is perceptive, vitally interested in the services provided by the health care organization, and readily critical of problems that might occur in the delivery of services. The organization that is vigilant with respect to customer/patient's needs and meets them effectively will enjoy long-term success.

Leaders who embrace the ethical tenet of customer commitment understand that the most important aspect of the health care mission is the provision of top-notch care and keep that tenet as a top priority in all work-related activities. They recognize that their livelihood and professional standing depend largely on their ability to contribute to the provision of high-quality health care service to those in need.

Some positive actions that demonstrate strong commitment begin with the supervisor and manager, both of whom are positioned to determine the effect of all work activity on the delivery of service. Managers realize that their departments are not autonomous entities within the organization, that in fact their roles and those of the departments they supervise relate directly to customer/patient satisfaction. For example, the pharmacy manager realizes that the quick and efficient preparation and delivery of prescriptions is key to the perception of organizational competency. Likewise, the parking lot supervisor who is understanding in the handling of visitor requests for parking is not abrupt to an individual who might be visiting a loved one in dire medical condition is also a living example of a health care professional who has a high degree of commitment.

Conscientious leaders will ask customer/patients questions that might help improve service delivery. Or they might review customer/patient relations information and guest relations data to see the relative effect their department has on the overall perception of customer/patient satisfaction.

Taking the process one step further, managers might talk to department employees, who can offer a wealth of information on activities and approaches to maximize customer/patient satisfaction. Professional journals can provide ideas on how higher commitment levels are achieved in other organizations. The most vital ethical mission of a health care organization—in fact, the one facet that makes the health care organization unique—is to determine critical customer/patient needs relative to basic human health and well-being. In this context the customer/patient drives the organization, not vice versa. The savvy manager ensures that the individuals working in his or her sphere of influence understand this fact as well.

Progressive managers might instill staff respect for and dedication to customer/patient service in a variety of fashions. First, they might have frequent meetings within the department to discuss commitment and different ways to build it into the daily routine. Second, in conjunction with the human resources department, they might have employees undertake a guest relations or customer/patient relations program, which not only will maximize their awareness of the needs of the customer/patient but also provide some practical methods to heighten departmental effectiveness in this area. Third, the manager might hold up as models of excellence the behavior of key staff members who have taken actions that significantly increased the department's effectiveness in this area. By rewarding these individuals (giving them bonuses or days off, for example), the manager is sending a clear message to all members of the organization about the importance of commitment. Simultaneously, other staff members are being motivated.

Forthright Tactics

The health care professional must conduct business honestly and fairly. Therefore, applying forthright tactics in every aspect of operation and business conduct is paramount. Essentially this means drawing on solid business standards and sound approaches to carry out assigned job duties and organizational responsibilities. The progressive manager, concerned as much with the means of performing a given assignment as with the end result, ensures that all action taken is ethical and aboveboard and takes into account the virtues of fairness and justice.

The health care professional who is perceived as an honest, steady player by pertinent organizational parties embraces forthright tactics as a normal method of operation; actions taken generally will not cause problems in the future or suffer negative repercussion. He or she can be counted on for ethical action and therefore will be a long-term contributor to the organization's progress. As a community member, his or her actions on the job serve to advertise the type of culture and business approach embraced by the health care organization.

Certain negative actions run counter to the principle of forthright tactics. For example, an individual interested only in results may be tempted to sacrifice method for outcome, running the risk of creating situations that can prove embarrassing to the organization. Negative actions can include improper use of financial resources, budget abuse, or employee overutilization. Each one of these actions can spell long-term trouble—funds shortages or high employee turnover, for example. Some managers may practice selective business ethics; that is, they may use sound business tactics only when convenient. The health care professional who does not have the courage of conviction and strength of character to use forthright tactics consistently may eventually fall under suspicion by subordinates and superiors alike, causing others to question whether he or she has the organization's best interests at heart.

Professional Liberty

Professional liberty has specific relevance for the executive or manager in a successful health care organization. As a business norm, *professional liberty* alludes to an individual who encourages each staff member to practice his or her trade in an environment that fosters independence. The progressive executive motivates team members to attain a high degree of professional acumen and a superlative level of competence and confidence. This manager realizes that human resources are the most important commodity a health care organization has. In looking beyond financial assets and physical resources, this leader views well-trained and highly motivated personnel to be the hallmark of the organization's success. By promoting professional liberty among staff, and by encouraging and facilitating their professional and technical growth, the manager helps the entire organization and upgrades the health care business in general.

Delegation is a primary tool for encouraging professional liberty. The manager who delegates appropriately and effectively uses a powerful developmental strategy. For example, by giving staff members work assignments they relish, can learn from, and master, the manager not only fosters growth but enhances motivation and competence. To delegate efficiently, the manager must know the strengths and limitations of each staff member as well as how strong his or her desire is to succeed. The manager should gather evidence to form a frame of reference relative to each individual's performance, promotability, and long-term potential, as demonstrated in the case study in chapter 8. These data will help the manager effect a system for promoting professional liberty with respect to each team member.

In another sense, a proponent of professional liberty is able to work smoothly with professionals from other departments in matrix management situations. *Matrix management* is a "custom-designed" approach to problem solving in which professionals from various technical areas form a work team to address a designated objective. The value-driven manager allows team members to bring to the equation their specific level of expertise, viewpoints, and suggestions. The host manager will share information with team members as needed and be a willing participant in their professional development scheme and in the attainment of work objectives.

This manager will optimize every opportunity to hone the skills of subordinates and assist them in reaching their highest professional potential. By acquiring a frame of reference for each subordinate in terms of performance, promotability, and potential, the manager will have a working knowledge of how best to implement a development plan tailored for each subordinate.

Quality

With the current proliferation of quality control and organizational quality programs in the health care training and development realm, most managers and executives are acutely aware of the need for quality. This section examines the quality perspective as a fundamental factor in the overall category of business norms.

Health care professionals who incorporate quality as part of the business norm strategy seek to apply the highest possible quality standards to all work performed by themselves as well as by their subordinates. Managers are intolerant of needless waste of resources, second-rate effort, inferior work production, or inferior customer/patient service. Quality, like all of the values discussed in this chapter, is not only a business dynamic but also an ethical one. Failure to adhere to high standards of quality represents an unethical breach of confidence between the customer/patient and the organization.

Individuals who set forth high standards of quality and incorporate them ethically into business norms set parameters on standards for performance goals as well as for the evaluation of individual employee performance. They are circumspect in determining what their employees can contribute yet unrelenting in encouraging them to accomplish these goals.

These individuals will also initiate and support departmental quality control and quality assurance programs that are encouraged by the organization. Furthermore, they will apply a quality control program within their organization or their particular department. This means using numerical indicators during a performance evaluation to assess the quality of work performed. The amount of time or money saved, an increase in the amount of work performed (such as more invoices processed per day), or a decrease in percentages of employee turnover, unfilled staffing vacancies, billing errors, and the like are all factors which relate to individual quality, and in turn, overall organizational effectiveness. These factors are discussed in more detail in chapter 6.

The manager who does not value quality will always look for the quickest route to an action conclusion, as opposed to the most effective route in terms of quality output. Integrity of action will be lacking, and a premium will be placed on completing the action as opposed to ensuring the quality of the completed product. This unfortunate priority will be evidenced in the focus on quantitative numbers as opposed to quality indicators. For example, an action might have been completed in the shortest time, but in the process the very quality issues that underlie the need for action may have been neglected. That is, if a hospital accounts receivable clerk reduced the time involved in collecting a payment but in the process reduced the actual amount of money collected, quality was sacrificed to quantity.

Social Awareness

The final business norm for value-driven health care management is social awareness. Because of the unique relationship between health care and societal dynamics, the manager must be committed to understanding the relevance of key social issues to the provision of high-quality health care. Not only is this smart business, it is also an ethical responsibility. A health care professional with a strong social awareness possesses a frame of reference in terms of how social issues affect the health care business—for example, demographics that affect the organization's customer/patient population. Aware managers can draw from this knowledge to help provide top-quality service to the community.

A socially aware manager will use a variety of sources to gather information on key sociological issues related to the delivery of health care services. These might include media reports that examine how the general public perceives key medical issues and health care dynamics. For example, the health care manager who was unaware of the nation's sensitivity to malpractice and the AIDS crisis in 1988 was in fact derelict in his or her ethical responsibilities to customer/patients. The same responsibility applies locally.

Key social concerns include employment, education, local politics, and ecology. For example, jobs are a central focus in a community; therefore, prominent employers influence the customer/patient population. Education bears on the level of communication that exists between a health care organization and a customer/patient. Political action within the area might have a profound effect on the customer community and in turn the local health care organization. For example, if politicians zone a particular piece of real estate for industrial development, expansion of the local population might occur. Ecological issues—toxic spills or leaks, high ozone indexes, pesticide poisoning—can have severe physical effects on the population, which may mean emergency treatment at the health care facility. The experienced health care professional goes beyond demographics in terms of assessing key issues of social awareness and looks at the various attitudes, likely outlooks, and widely held perceptions of the customer community. These give clues on how the conduct of health care operations in the community might be affected.

A health care professional, particularly at the executive level, must anticipate trends that will affect future delivery of health care services to the community. The current ongoing attention given to the abortion issue is a key example in this regard in that it has become a major moral and ethical issue for health care professionals to wrestle with. Americans— male and female—are vitally interested in how political action and sociological change will affect legislation of this issue. Resolution of the abortion issue is bound to have profound effects on the health care community; the health care professional who demonstrates social awareness and compassion will anticipate how the outcome will affect teens, single women, and the families of those involved in the specific abortion cases.

Again from an executive perspective, the savvy health care leader will weave his or her frame of social awareness into practice as part of an employee relations program. Specifically, this means promoting understanding that the actions of the local community affect the members of the organization, members who live in the very community served by the health care organization. For example, following the dynamics of a local political campaign and how it will affect employees and growth of a health care organization is one facet of employee relations. Or, if a manufacturer shuts down, the prudent health care executive will re-examine the organization's benefit package to assist its employees who have family members affected by the plant shutdown. If a social issue bears on the health care organization, the executive's ethical responsibility to the community and to the organization's members is to take appropriate, proactive, and effective action.

As indicated earlier in this section, the smart executive will respond to national social issues with appropriate strategies in customer/patient services and employee relations. If a national trend demands a new or expanded service, the successful health care organization will respond quickly. Examples include "Smoke-Out" programs, which responded to protests against the harmful effect of tobacco, and stress management, which many hospitals have capitalized on by offering community outreach programs. The smart health care executive will use this level of social awareness not only as a business opportunity but an ethical service to the customer/patient community.

☐ Executive Principles

Executive principles include dependability, exemplary conduct, optimization of resources, positive power, and visibility.

Dependability

Dependability is defined as the ability and willingness to make executive decisions, take leadership action, and set organizational policies and standards that are consistent with the attainment of ethical excellence in the provision of high-quality health care services. In short, it charges the executive with the responsibility to take action as needed in a sound, consistent fashion. This is vitally important not only to the executive but to those who must follow his or her leadership. Lack of consistency or continuity of action can lead subordinates to lose faith in the executive's quality of decision making. Dependability is an ethical standard because it deals with the heart of executive responsibility (decision making).

An executive who pragmatically embraces the value of dependability can be relied on to consider all viable viewpoints prior to making a decision. He or she will solicit the opinions of subordinates and experts.

Also considered will be the viewpoints of others who might be affected. Once the decision is made, the executive will take full responsibility for the outcome.

Implicit in dependability is continuity from one related action to another. Dependable executives maintain a high level of consistency in their actions, an aspect of management known as progressive development. When one decision acts as a building block to yet another decision in a related action, this helps to create a sense of direction and overall mission to all in the chain of command. The executive who subscribes to the concept of progressive development realizes that the overall mission of a successful health care organization is to provide superior health care. In a general sense, all decisions made keep the customer/patient in mind and lead from one action to the other toward accomplishing that end. In a specific sense, all the manager's actions are interrelated, so that staff members and subordinates have a clear idea not only of what the general mission of the organization is but, more important, what specific programs are being pursued to accomplish that mission.

Exemplary Conduct

A health care executive who embraces exemplary conduct as part of the everyday work routine maintains an organizational leadership role and a presence in the community that reflects a humanistic commitment, positive outlook, and creditable desire to provide stellar service to those in need. In essence, this individual serves as an example of professionalism both to organizational members and to the customer/patient community. Executives who embrace exemplary conduct set standards to be emulated through all layers of the organization. For example, executive conduct, both on the job and away from the workplace, does not make for good gossip material. These leaders do not engage in activities that might lead other staff members to believe they are social schizophrenics. A social schizophrenic is typified by appropriate and ethical behavior on the job, but away from the workplace he or she engages in activities that might arouse suspicion about his or her true ethical composition. In small communities in particular, when an individual has a *proven* reputation for spending a lot of time in taverns or has a number of DWI convictions, for example, his or her ethical behavior during working hours is sure to come under suspicion.

Executives who demand high ethical standards of conduct from their staffs without overstepping legal boundaries positively execute a system of exemplary conduct. That is, they expect their subordinates and staff members to ascribe to the same ethical approach to work that they do. Finally, their on-the-job behavior incorpor⁻ ˙s all of the ethical standards discussed in the first six chapters of thi ⃰ ⅛k.

Optimization of Resources

The executive principle of optimization of resources is demonstrated by a health care leader who utilizes all available financial, operational, and human resources to their fullest potential in the interest of efficiency and effectiveness. His or her leadership style encourages maximum contributions from all members of the organization. In the current health care business arena it is imperative that executives and managers make the most of their available resources. With shrinking revenues and a changing customer/patient base, medical facilities of all types must avoid wasting and misusing their resources. Consequently, the importance of optimization of resources is underscored not only as a managerial directive but an ethical imperative.

The health care executive who uses resources optimally understands the technical and professional strengths of all the organization's players. Therefore this individual can delegate activities among all workers. Doing so minimizes the need for additional human, operational, or financial resources not in the budget. For example, if the director of an MIS (management information system) knows about the untapped potential of a computer operator, it may not be necessary to hire temporary personnel or to subcontract a smaller MIS firm to accomplish a specific objective.

The hallmark of an executive who optimizes resources fully considers efficiency of action as well as effectiveness of outcome. This means the executive always weighs the time and money expenditure of a particular project against the quality of outcome. If this means using two individuals to perform one job in half the time with twice the productivity, the manager will make that call, keeping in mind the imperative to exhaust available resources. A side benefit of this mandate is that workers will be encouraged to try new methods and different approaches to accomplishing an objective—a venture that might prove more cost-effective and time-efficient.

Resourceful executives refuse to be daunted by the lack of an "ideal" supply of resources. Rather, they will try to use available resources innovatively. *Innovation* is defined in this context as the ability to use existing resources in a novel, more productive manner.

Finally, individuals who optimize resources understand that human resources are the most important and often the most challenging to manage. They will seek to learn as much as possible about creative ways of motivating subordinates and inspiring their creative contributions, and making optimum use of all their resources. Making the most of the resources at hand, as opposed to wishing for resources that are not available, is the hallmark of an effective executive in this regard.

Positive Power

Positive power is the ability to use the offices of leadership as a charter to serve others—most important the customer/patient community—by displaying competency of management and a spirit of professionalism in every business endeavor. The executive who properly uses positive power never abuses his or her power of office or ignores responsibility in fulfilling an executive charter to the health care organization.

Power is an important executive tool in any business arena. Power facilitates decision making, influences the lives of all members of the organization, and warrants the future progress of the organization. Proper use of power inspires confidence and commitment from all people related to the organization; misuse of power creates suspicion, mistrust, and ultimate failure of the organization.

Health care executives who employ positive power as an ongoing ethical strategy exercise a good balance between power and humility; they do not let organizational power "go to their heads." That is, they do not become autocratic, insensitive, or hurtful in the execution of their responsibilities. They graciously—and gratefully—accept opinions and advice from others and do not feel that they "know it all." They realize that executive privilege is exactly that: a privilege and the result of hard work and career progression, not a preordained right.

The executive exercising power in a positive way has a clear vision of what the organization is about and what it should accomplish, both in the long term and the short term. He or she can inspire and challenge others to share that vision and embrace its objectives fully. Executive power can motivate 10 different staff members in 10 different ways toward the mission, taking time to understand their desires and to rally efforts toward progress on the job and contribution to the organization's objectives.

Powerful leaders do not issue ultimatums; they are nonmanipulative and nonthreatening. Power is not used to breed favoritism among or between the staff. Nor should power be the excuse for unwarranted or rash decisions or decisions that are not pertinent to the accomplishment of goals—for example, "pulling rank" to rearrange furniture in a work group merely because the manager wants to exercise authority. This will only encourage subversion and failure to take the manager's direction seriously, in that this behavior is not perceived as being well intentioned or in the interest of organizational performance.

An executive who takes advantage of an inordinate amount of personal "perks" also abuses power. Whether it is a personalized parking spot or excessive time off, such perks communicate that the executive is "better" than others in the chain of command. Respect dictated by a power-crazed executive is not true respect, and a fundamental breakdown of command will occur.

Leaders are self-demanding in all aspects of their roles, which in turn encourages the same spirit of commitment from others. They do not constantly rely on negative motivation as a primary strategy in getting tasks accomplished but use their power of management to formulate meaningful strategies and ethical tactics that serve to fulfill organizational goals and desired ends. They do not discipline workers without cause or manage by intimidation—as often occurs with managers who are insecure in their work roles or not intelligent or ethical enough to realize that long-term motivation is best facilitated by challenging and creative direction.

An executive competent in every area of responsibility, from technical aspects to fiscal control to people management, is likely to use power positively as a progressive strategy. This person has a high level of confidence, which will assist in providing spirited management, and uses the power as a tool in the administration or assignment of responsibilities and in the management of relegated resources. Positive power employed correctly is the most effective, long-lasting, progressive style of management.

Undercutting the authority of others is an example of negative power. This could include making decisions for supervisors instead of letting them make their own decisions or (as seen) making decisions not in the purview of assigned executive responsibilities. Both actions demonstrate lack of faith in supervisors and managers assigned to the executive, and both are demoralizing as well as demotivating. It also shows lack of ethical commitment to management's development.

Visibility

By actions and presence in all business situations—particularly in tough circumstances—a health care executive can maintain high visibility and keep his or her commitment to the organization's mission in the forefront. Examples of this include presenting useful ideas based on sound concepts of health care management when participating in meetings and conferences, and being willing to take the lead and make an impact on meetings, which help determine important outcomes to the organization. Furthermore, high-profile executives are willing to explain the rationale behind tough decisions they have made. They can resolve difficult organizational problems innovatively and (as noted) maintain solid responsibility for their actions.

Visibility reinforces the notion that they are approachable and ever ready to help subordinates or staff members who need their advice. They help to encourage and support clear-cut ethical action among subordinates and superiors and do all they can to help facilitate ethical, sound management practices on the part of their peers and coworkers. They constantly challenge their managers and supervisors to take a firm stand on tough issues and to back up those positions with solid data and rationale.

The visibility directive demands that executives let people know where they stand on major issues and make it clear that their stance is based on the best data available at the time and is taken with the best interest of all concerned in mind. Their ideas or positions on key organizational matters are not left to conjecture or guesswork. Up-front leaders are perceived by workers as people who can be relied on to do the right thing in new situations.

Visible executives are the first on the scene in dire circumstances, their commitment to the organization never waivers, and they are easy to find in tough situations that demand "something extra."

The executive who is nowhere to be found when things get tough will never educate players as to why a specific action was taken or a certain position advocated. This elusive leader does not want to "face the heat," which is typical of one who lacks self-confidence or who possesses a disproportionate desire to save face no matter what. Such an individual is always around to take the cheers but never to hear the boos.

☐ Practical Applications

The following ideas may serve as a starting point for incorporating the principles of value-driven management into your work setting:

1. Review each of the four categories of performance values for relevance to your work activities as well as to those of your staff.
2. Review and be able to explain the 20 values as they relate to your work role and to your subordinates.
3. Incorporate the values into your selection and hiring practices, supplemented with the information and interview questions in appendix A.
4. Use the values as part of training and development efforts for employees and professional staff.
5. Use the values as discussion points in board retreats and other activities with the board of directors.
6. Augment the criteria for each value with your own perceptions and "success factors" regarding value-driven management.
7. Utilize the values to conduct an organizational assessment of a new work group or sphere of responsibility.
8. Discuss the importance of each value and supplemental criteria with each of your employees separately so as to gain a fuller application of the material.

9. Add these values to your performance evaluation process, as demonstrated by section II of the sample value-driven performance evaluation plan in appendix B. The subject of performance planning and evaluation is treated in more detail in chapters 6, 7, and 8.
10. Incorporate these values into your mission and values statement and related activities.

Progressive Motivational Strategies

As specified in the preceding two chapters, a set of leadership princi-ples and organizational values should guide the health care manager's daily administrative strategies. In an effective organization, the every-day use of such principles and values is essential to maintaining work-place harmony and progressive performance. However, an additional dimension of management—employee motivation—is necessary to apply these executive principles and values to the workplace in a meaningful and productive fashion.

This chapter examines an array of motivational strategies that, when combined with the principles and values in chapters 2 and 3, constitute a more comprehensive approach to progressive health care management. The motivators discussed in this chapter (chosen from among the 50 motivators described in appendix C) illustrate a process for enhancing ability to motivate the reporting staff.

The use of various motivational strategies has been a topic of indus-trial psychology research since its inception, which is generally credited to Abraham Maslow. Maslow's simple and oft-cited premise—the human need for self-esteem, security, and affiliation—is still at the root of many theories and practicums in vogue today. The author's experience has found that a roster of about 50 motivators is used by a successful health care manager or executive. These motivators fall into categories based on five characteristics:

1. Environmental and organization-driven
2. Management-controlled
3. Individual
4. Job-related
5. Jointly established

This chapter explores some sample motivators from each category, their potential implementation in the reader's arsenal of motivational

techniques, and their relevance to the leadership principles and underlying values of progressive health care management. In addition to sum-
marizing each motivator, appendix C provides work sheets for planning
your own enhancement strategies.

☐ Environmental and Organization-Driven Motivators

To understand the importance of skillful motivation of health care workers, from housekeeper to CEO, it is essential first to consider why workers leave one position for another. Think of all of the reasons used by
a disgruntled employee upon resigning from a position: "This organization doesn't seem the same anymore," "I don't feel as though I'm growing anymore," "I'm not sure what we're trying to achieve here anymore,"
"I wonder who really is in charge here." Almost all of these reasons
revolve around a lack of motivation or the presence of de-motivating factors. For every reason why a good employee leaves, there usually is an
equal and opposite reason why a good employee stays. With that in
mind, an examination of motivators must originate with those managed
and mandated by the organization and its environment.

Organizational Design

Controlled mainly by the board of directors and the chief executive officer
(CEO), health care organizational design refers to the organization's structure and reporting relationships, which in turn reflect the CEO's style
of control and its presence throughout the organization. Ideally, the
design should encourage maximum interchange of ideas and information among all employees, in addition to an ability to respond quickly
to work requests and to approve necessary actions in a timely fashion.

As indicated in table 4-1, the CEO's power and ability to influence
the work of a given organization is related closely to the type of organization established by the board of directors and the main administration. The three types of organization are the autocracy, the pyramid, and
the participative democracy. Each type will dictate a set of influence
processes used by a leader. For example, in an autocratic style of control, chief management may use intimidation –"do this or else"– and stress
the dire consequences of not complying with an organizational directive or work objective. Tradition can be also used as an influence process
by demanding a certain mode of work behavior because "that's the way
it's always been done."

The pyramid organization influences employees with two types of
faith, that is, with a psychological investment as encouraged and inspired
by the organization. The first type is *blind faith*, with which members

Table 4-1. Power and Influence Schemes by Organization Type

Organization Type	Power and Influence Scheme	Characteristics
1. Autocracy	• Total executive control • Fear and coercion as motivators • Dictatorship decisions • No midmanagement participation	• Highly structured corporate culture, little innovation, limited reaction to change, restricted communication
2. Pyramid	• Balance among the organization, departments, and individuals • Organizational progress is key motivator	• Clear assignment of duties and responsibilities; delegation and independent judgment are valued
3. Participative democracy	• "All for one and one for all" • The individual is the *most* important organizational component • Everyone in the organization is encouraged to present an opinion about everything	• Tendency toward process over product; communication and input given higher priority than action and efficiency in some cases

of the organization absolutely believe in its objectives and render their support of those objectives with little or no discussion or arbitration. In essence, they believe everything required of them is for the good of the organization and, ultimately, for their own good. This allows the pyramid organization to maintain a strong sense of command, and in fact uses a very structured and sound chain of command.

The other type of faith elicited by a pyramid organization is *rational faith*. The employee is allowed to make a considered decision whether to follow the leadership and directives of the organization based on individual understanding and commitment to the organizational directives and mission. Rational faith differs from blind faith only in that the employee feels as though he or she is a part of the decision-making process, albeit a very minor contributor.

The third type of organizational design, participative democracy, is often called "management by committee" by many industrial psychologists. In this type of design, organizational power and influence is determined by one of two influence processes: rational agreement or joint determination.

To build *rational agreement,* the leader incorporates employee suggestions on work objectives into group plans, and rational agreement is augmented by the understanding and ratification of plans by the rest of the group. For example, consider the chief financial officer (CFO) of a major metropolitan hospital who has the objective of completing an audit of all the hospital operations. Under the scheme of rational agreement, the auditor will prepare a plan of action (which includes the investigation of various records, delegation of assignments to subordinates, and distribution of work to all members of the staff), then present this plan to the staff and encourage their input to the basic structure of the plan. In doing so, the CFO encourages participation and by doing so will likely get ideas and suggestions that will add to the plan's effectiveness. At the conclusion of this process, ownership is shared by all members of the CFO's staff, and each participant feels as though the plan is truly "ours," as opposed to being "his" or "hers."

Joint determination in a participative democracy is the type of influence process that generated the phrase "management by committee." In utilizing this process, the aforementioned CFO would allow staff participation in determining why the audit should be completed, how it might be completed, what resources should be used, which is the most appropriate method to use in completing the audit, and so forth. Although the motivation factor in this case might be shared ownership by members, in the long run this scheme becomes less motivating as action becomes stalled and minor details are deliberated endlessly. This method also opens the door for the more verbose members of the staff to suggest opinion after opinion, with little regard for relevance.

It is the contention of this author, as well as many other industrial psychologists, that rational agreement is to be preferred over joint determination as a method of motivation in a participative democracy.

Given the potential shortcomings of a participative democracy, most experts agree that the pyramid structure is best for motivating employees. In a pyramid arrangement, employees can see where the next progressive career step is, who's in charge of their work destiny, and how an actual chain of command controls the intended success of their organization. Nevertheless, the pyramid structure should accommodate some form of rational agreement so that leaders garner support from subordinates as well as develop a certain depth of vision in each employee according to his or her specific area of expertise and responsibility. This also entitles the employee to a measure of self-direction, which allows a cohesive work unit to become even more galvanized in its work and sense of purpose.

Affiliation

Another environmental and organization-driven motivator is affiliation, the sense of belonging that the employee has relative to the organization and its objectives. Most members of the health care community, from the nursing home industry to the larger metropolitan medical centers, feel a strong sense of pride in their professional endeavors if they are working for a successful organization that is respected throughout the community. Picking up on the original Maslow theme, they feel a strong sense of positive motivation because they are affiliated with a winning enterprise and a successful venture. Moreover, they feel that they are dedicating their professional lives to an organization that pursues excellence in providing needed health care.

This sense of affiliation can be made stronger by planning activities that underscore the employees' positive feeling of membership in the progressive organization, one that has the "right stuff." Such activities might include steering committee assignments and organizationwide social activities. Other methods of underscoring this sense of affiliation can include visible expressions of membership, such as employee uniforms, stationery, and tote bags with the organization's logo.

Social Interaction

Another environment-based motivator is social interaction. Considering once again the relationship between the reasons for employee turnover and the importance of positive motivation, the comment "the people at this organization aren't my type of people" is a powerful reminder of how important social interaction on the job is to employee motivation. Because the organization regulates and sets standards for the type of employees hired, and the successful organization ascribes to a set profile for employee selection and performance, this indeed becomes an organizational/environmental issue.

The successful health care organization determines a set of acceptable ethical behaviors, work personalities, and team orientation factors that prescribe the type of individual it hires, develops, and rewards. Although personality nuances and personal quirks exist within every organization, workers with sound ethical standards, the ability to make significant contributions to the work group, and a desire to grow as professionals are the backbone of the successful health care organization. Leaders must weigh these factors in their hiring process to ensure that social interaction on the job is grounded by a commonality of purpose and dedication. Chapter 3 and appendix A examined the personal values, humanistic standards, business norms, and executive principles that characterize outstanding members of the progressive health care team.

Mission Identification

Related to social interaction is the motivational factor of mission identification. All successful health care organizations design a mission statement that communicates organizational objectives and values as well as a commitment to provide high-quality health care services to a designated community. The mission statement is disseminated and reinforced throughout the entire organization.

A leader in the health care environment must use the power of his or her position to ensure that the organizational mission is perceived as being creditable and relevant to all employees. Employees in a high-stress health care environment must feel day in and day out that their organization is dedicated to the provision of health care for those in need as well as to an assortment of ethical standards. Whereas the mission of a stockbroker firm or other financial institution might primarily be to make money, with employees who are dedicated to the same end, the primary mission in a health care environment—and thus that of its employees—is more intangible and complex. Therefore, it is essential to ensure that a strong mission statement is in place, understood by all members of the organization, and seen as more than just lip service to an ideal. This is accomplished by the visible, dependable, and exemplary conduct exhibited by the organization's leaders.

Organizational Development

The employee who cites lack of professional growth as a reason for leaving has been victimized by an organization that failed to provide a progressive professional skills development strategy. As will be discussed in later chapters of this book, a good development program must be installed along with a good performance evaluation program in order to communicate clearly the development opportunities available to each employee. Furthermore, each supervisor must make a concerted effort to provide development opportunities on the job so that each employee can steadily enhance his or her technical and professional capabilities. Delegation strategies, training programs, and in-service programs are examples of methods toward this end. Good employees want to be challenged not only by their current work roles but by experiences that will allow them to learn more about their job, expand their professional responsibilities, and learn more about the health care profession in general.

Tangible Benefits

An effective development program is incorporated as part of a larger motivational strategy, that of providing competitive tangible benefits. In addition to basic wages and monetary bonuses, tangible benefits might include life insurance, medical insurance, meal programs, and/or parking. Educational development opportunities are certainly part of a tangible benefit program and therefore vital to employee motivation. In light of the increased competition for skilled health care workers, the successful organization must provide as many tangible employee benefits as its budget will allow. The case study in chapter 10 includes some additional ideas for tangible benefits. For purposes of this discussion, the following is a checklist of tangible motivators used by today's progressive health care executives:

- "Pay-for-performance" compensation
- Life insurance
- Comprehensive health insurance
- Dental insurance
- Bonus plans
- Day-care facilities
- Tuition reimbursement
- Employee purchase programs
- Social activities offered at reduced rates
- Savings programs
- Parking accommodations
- Meal discounts
- Vacations with pay
- Shift differentials
- Holiday/weekend extra pay
- On-site accreditation programs
- Full (100 percent) dependent insurance coverage

Security and Stability

An employee's sense of job and income security stems from the organization's fiscal stability and ability to maintain profitability under changing conditions. A sense of stability is developed when turbulent change in the external environment does not drastically affect the overall organization and when internal change does not affect individual work roles or personal growth and progress. In that change is a necessary evil within most health care organizations, the facility that responds well to change and strives to turn negative change into positive change communicates a message of organizational stability to its members. Good stability within an organization in turn provides good security for each job classification.

With the plethora of facility closings, reorganizations, and buyouts, the organization that can provide at least a semblance of organizational *stability* and individual *security* addresses these two motivational needs of its employees. Once again, the health care manager who can demonstrate that he or she (1) is in charge and is concerned about each employee's welfare and (2) can be relied on to make decisions that affect the organization positively during periods of change is the conduit for these motivators. (The management of change is discussed in more detail in chapter 5.)

Usage of Various Motivators

The intelligent health care manager understands the various dimensions of environmental and organization-driven motivators and their impact on each employee. To assist the reader in utilizing these motivators, appendix C presents work sheets for identifying:

- Pertinent examples of individuals (or departments) who have demonstrated high levels of motivation for each motivating factor
- Potential targets for motivation, whether individuals on the reporting staff or entire departments within the organization
- Choice of strategy for enhancing the motivation of reporting staff or departments

By reviewing these motivators periodically in checklist fashion, and by implementing strategies that address the needs of individual employees or departments, the organization can foster high productivity and solid performance from all personnel through strong mission identification and strong commitment to the organization and its operational precepts.

☐ Management-Controlled Motivators

Several motivating factors are controlled by individual managers, supervisors, and department heads relative to the manner in which they assign work, provide direction and inspiration for work completion, and set general job conduct standards.

The Fun Quotient

As a motivator *fun* can be defined as the degree of enjoyment that an employee finds in pursuing job tasks. Most organizational development specialists and industrial psychologists agree that an individual worker in any profession who enjoys at least 60 percent of the job responsibilities is well motivated. A manager who makes every effort to present an enjoyable work climate, challenging job objectives, and a sense of positive spirit for work goals will maximize the "fun quotient" in each job. Obviously, due to the nature of the health care mission, not all circumstances within a health care setting are fun or even enjoyable. It is equally evident that some aspects of a job description may be more enjoyable than others. Basically these are the activities in which the employee is highly interested and proficient. The manager must seek to build the job description, and center the employee's activities, on these more enjoyable characteristics.

Work Interest

Similar to the fun quotient, 60 percent of an employee's average work-day is applied to the activity related to the employee's genuine work interests. In other words, if administrative tasks, meetings, answering the phone, and other relatively uninteresting tasks exceed 40 percent of the workday, the employee will soon become de-motivated. In applying the executive principle of optimization of resources, the intelligent and introspective health care manager will strive to determine the employee's keenest source of work interest, professional pride, and technical expertise to center a job description on the most motivating aspects. This, balanced with the organization's need to have employees undertake some necessary but mundane tasks, will determine a solution of maximum motivation relative to work interests. The manager should engage the employee in conversations that focus specifically on job design and implement a series of management controls that ensure the completion of mundane tasks as well as the steady provision of more interesting job responsibilities.

Achievement and Recognition

A fundamental aspect of the motivation of any individual, in health care or any other profession, is that of achievement. Organizational members are encouraged to aspire and work toward their respective highest level of performance and are provided with the support and resources to reach it. Without measurable achievement within a work role, an employee feels as though he or she is "going nowhere," which is an oft-cited reason for resignation from a position. The manager of a particular department, or an executive of an entire organization, is in charge of providing opportunities for employee achievement. One strategy to demonstrate achievement publicly is the implementation of an "employee of the month" program or other forms of recognition.

Achievement and recognition must go hand in hand; the employee who gains good job results should be recognized through promotion, wage raises, and any other such "strokes." Failure to reach the performance potential that one is capable of breeds frustration and distrust of the organization. Lack of recognition for achievements breeds discontent and a sense of being unappreciated.

Independence

Independence is the relative degree of autonomy given to each employee in the pursuit of attaining set goals and objectives, as well as the amount of input allowed from the employee in setting those goals. The degree of job independence an employee needs is related directly to the employee's expertise in a given work role, his or her work personality, and the type of job undertaken.

Depending on their personality traits, some employees enjoy a strong sense of independence and need little direction from the manager once goals and desired outcomes are understood. Others need more direction and thus appreciate a high degree of managerial visibility and interaction. Each manager must ascertain the level of independence desired by each employee and, perhaps most important, the level of independence needed to motivate the employee to maximum productivity.

Independence is another tool for optimizing resources and requires introspection on the part of the manager to know not only each employee's strengths, weaknesses, and potential but also the level of independence desired. A strongly independent employee can quickly be de-motivated by a manager who has a proclivity for "peeking over the employee's shoulder." On the other hand, a new or inexperienced employee can feel alienation and lack of direction from a manager who mistakenly gives too much independence.

Change

Another management-controlled motivator, change within the workplace, causes employee response to new dimensions in the workplace—for example, increased demands for output, shifting objectives, the assimilation of new resources, and alterations in standards of performance. Some managers believe that a certain amount of change is good in order to keep employees "on their toes." Other managers believe the opposite— that a steady flow of direction and a sense of reliable supervision is a good motivator.

Depending on your organization and its individual work roles, the introduction of change can be good or bad. Work activity and the nature of individual work roles determine the degree of change and how it might affect individual employees. Most health care managers believe a minimum of change is required for the successful motivation of hourly employees, whose job descriptions are somewhat staid, whereas executives believe they and their managers need a certain extent of change in order to be intellectually challenged.

Work activity, job description, and, most important, the needs of the organization should all be taken into account when considering change within the workplace as a motivating factor. It must be added that too much change can wear out the adaptability of any worker at any particular level within the organization; not enough change can bring about boredom.

Reward Systems

A system of rewards is a set of procedures for compensating outstanding performance. Rewards can be monetary and nonmonetary. Each manager must determine what reward his or her respective charges desire from their work productivity.

As demonstrated later in this chapter, most employees desire a certain living wage in addition to other benefits. There are several hidden rewards, however, that can be awarded by a manager to individual employees for their work efforts. By combining some of the motivators cited in this section, the manager might provide opportunity for a rewarding experience. For example, the employee might be given a chance to work on a particular project he or she finds highly enjoyable and interesting (fun quotient + work interest) or to increase job responsibility (independence + change). Or a request for reassignment to another section or department might be granted (achievement and recognition + work interest + change). Yet another reward might be to invite the employee to participate in an activity that can further professional development and growth (achievement and recognition + independence + change).

Attainment of a positive reward is as effective as the "carrot or stick" method. A carrot for the workhorse was a reward for good work in the plow field; the whack of a stick, on the other hand, was a consequence for a job poorly done. In this vein, the progressive health care manager must look beyond monetary compensation for other "carrots" that motivate the employee.

☐ Individual Motivators

Just as each employee brings a set of skills and abilities to a health care organization, each employee also brings certain proclivities in terms of is motivating. This section reviews these individual motivators in the interest of providing a perspective for using them and understanding their impact on each employee's work output.

Money

The most prominent individual motivator is money. Many new-wave industrial psychologists deny that money is a motivator, maintaining that the short-term effects of a pay raise or a large salary are usually outweighed by work interest and other motivators discussed in this chapter. In the estimation of most health care managers, however, money is indeed a motivator; to most health care employees it is a measure of their professional value. For example, registered nurses and physical therapists who work in the United States or Canada know chapter and verse the pay scale and benefits for positions in their area. Therefore, if a worker's wage is below the norm, chances are he or she will be de-motivated and perform poorly. If his or her wage is in sync with or above the going rate, chances are that money will not be a de-motivator but a motivator—it may even be secondary to other motivators, such as work interest or work climate. Using wage scale data to adjust pay scales is essential for an institution to maintain a strong presence in this influential area.

Ego

As an individual motivator, ego is the barometer of self-esteem an individual brings to the workplace as measured by his or her feelings of self-worth and gratification that come from contributing to the workplace. From Maslow's theory and other precepts of industrial psychology, it is known that self-esteem is a major factor in the motivation of an individual in a work situation. An employee's ego and sense of self-esteem must be understood by the manager or executive and taken into account in providing direction and work objectives for the employee.

A common management technique is to appeal to the ego. For example, if a medical technician perceives himself as an expert in his field, the manager, in appealing to his ego, will often say, "As the expert in this field, you're the person we are relying on. . . ." In other words, the manager appeals to the prevailing factor of that individual's self-esteem to obtain the work result desired. Although this is a good short-term approach, the manager must incorporate all (or as many as possible) aspects of motivation to ensure that the employee is not being recognized at a rate that is disproportionate to other deserving members of the work group. The manager also must take care to ensure that the employee does not become egocentric or a megalomaniac in respect to the work role. This could breed a false sense of the employee's importance relative to the job characteristics and to the organization and, if not properly managed, could develop into creating a "superstar complex" around a particular individual. However, as a final consideration, each manager must look at the ego gratification desired by each employee and try to determine on an individual basis how best to address that need through tangible and intangible rewards and recognition within the job.

Authority

All health care professionals, regardless of their level within the organization, desire a certain amount of authority relative to their work position.

This authority can be granted in terms of how much decision-making power they hold, how much discretion they have in using a particular instrument or piece of equipment, or their authority over the general direction of their work and the control of resources relative to accomplishing work-related goals.

Good managers usually delegate authority commensurate with the responsibility required to complete a certain job. Some individuals, principally highly technical workers or hourly workers, want no authority or decision-making responsibilities. Most employees, however, want autonomy relative to their job description and aspects of their work not addressed within their manager's sphere of authority. The manager should convey faith in an individual and respect for his or her technical expertise and outline distinctly the degree of authority each individual has in a given work situation. This creates a sense of independence for the employee, good optimization of resources for the manager, and a guarantee that the individual will not overstep bounds in pursuing a work objective.

Satisfaction

The measure of work satisfaction varies from individual to individual within a health care organization. As a motivator, *satisfaction* can be defined as a feeling of self-fulfillment, which is reflected in daily contribution to the workplace and in the knowledge that that contribution is vital.

Some people are satisfied by giving a "good day's work for a good day's wage." Other well-meaning employees can often set their level of satisfaction at an unrealistically high rate of accomplishment. For example, if an individual does not accomplish a goal or objective in a day, he or she might not derive a strong sense of satisfaction from daily activities.

Starting with the interview process, a manager or executive should try to determine what level of satisfaction an individual is looking for in a given work role. Questions to ask during the interview might include:

- How do you feel your career has developed so far?
- Can you tell me about the best job you've had in health care?
- What type of satisfaction do you derive from your current job?
- What is your favorite thing about your last/current job?
- What parts of your job provide the greatest sense of satisfaction?
- What do you look for in your next health care position?

Employee satisfaction levels can be ascertained by asking them to respond to the following statements with "strongly agree," "agree," "neutral," "disagree," or "strongly disagree":

- I am satisfied with my current job role.
- I have the resources necessary to perform my job optimally.
- I am satisfied with my compensation level and benefit package.
- To my knowledge, most of my peers are satisfied with their work and the organization.
- I look forward to the future challenges presented by my job.

Supervisory Responsibilities

Supervisory responsibilities are often cited as an *organizational* motivator. However, some individuals are de-motivated by supervisory responsibilities, whereas others relish them as part of their job assignment. Supervisory responsibilities are often mistakenly limited to the supervision of other human resources, whereas supervision of physical, equipment, or financial resources can also be delegated to the individual by the organization. Individuals determine whether or not they want to take on these responsibilities before taking a job.

Therefore, the delegation of supervisory responsibilities is a largely individual motivator and must be understood by the manager and related to the work role as such. For example, if a laboratory technician is promoted into a supervisory role based on expertise as a laboratory technician, the manager risks bringing the oft-cited Peter principle into play. That is, although the individual is promoted on the basis of past performance, he or she may have been promoted into a level of incompetence as a supervisor. Perhaps the individual never wanted supervisory responsibilities or was never trained for such responsibilities. If an individual is truly motivated to supervise people or equipment, the manager must try to incorporate a development scheme that will eventually bring this person into a position of supervisory responsibilities commensurate with his or her motivational desires and needs.

Personal Growth

Each individual sets a certain level of personal growth that he or she expects a work role to provide. Some workers desire to be better communicators and people persons and have keen interpersonal skills and a knowledge of what makes others tick. Others look for professional growth on the job. Still others consider growth to be an attainment of management and supervisory skills.

Whatever the individual's needs for personal growth, they must be addressed within the job or he or she may resign, saying "I felt as though I stopped growing in that position." A proactive strategy is for the health care manager to converse during the performance evaluation about what growth an individual desires and how the manager might best provide that growth through work direction and professional goals and objectives.

Intangible Benefits

Intangible benefits, that is, nonmonetary job rewards, are highly valued by the individual and uniquely provided by the organization to meet a personal need or desire. Intangible benefits can include the following:

- Preferred geographic location of the health care organization
- Ease of traffic flow and other dynamics in getting to and from work
- Manageable stress within the workplace and in a given job
- Desirability of union or nonunion workplace
- Type of control exerted by management over employees on a given assignment or long-term project
- A growing organization with new facilities
- An older established organization with long-term links to the customer community
- An organization with a particular type of computer system or other technical or physical facilities
- Family members or close friends employed by the organization
- Degree of visibility the organization has within the customer/patient community
- Local environment in which the organization operates
- Perceived growth and development of the organization

All of these factors are potential individual motivators. During a performance evaluation in an employment interview a manager should try to determine what intangible benefits an employee is looking for. By evaluating the desirability of these intangible benefits, a manager is more likely to find a good, long-term match between employee and organization.

☐ Job-Related Motivators

Job-related motivators include the job description and job design, as well as other motivators stemming from the nature of the job itself.

Job Description

Any discussion of job-related motivators must begin with the job description provided by management to the individual health care employee. This tool describes major areas of ongoing job activity, including the content of everyday activities that comprise the majority of compensated performance and evaluated output. The job description should also contain the number of tasks and responsibilities the individual will undertake, and the criteria by which the employee will be ranked relative to performance.

In many successful organizations, the job description is reviewed annually, if not semiannually, by both the employee and the supervisor to ensure that its content is timely and meaningful. In doing so, the organization ensures that the employee is providing maximum effort while obtaining maximum opportunity for growth and development within the job. By including employees in ongoing maintenance of the job description, the organization ensures not only that the *breadth* of general responsibilities is ascribed to but also that the *depth* of individual potential and achievement is documented. Many employees leave an organization dissatisfied because they feel they never had an accurate job description, or they feel the way in which their performance was evaluated had little to do with the stated job description.

Job Design

Equally important to the job description is the design of the individual job. Job design is the structure of the particular work role, which includes lines of report, allocated resources, and avenues of communication. The latter includes the style and frequency of communication the individual has with others in the job.

As an example of how job design affects motivation, managers need to keep in mind that many individuals in health care, as well as in other industries, have what is commonly known as "phone phobia." They dislike using the phone, and often this level of discomfort manifests itself in inaccurate communication or misunderstood data being exchanged over the phone wires. For the employee with phone phobia, the demands of high levels of phone contact could become a de-motivator in a short period of time.

Therefore, the design of the job, that is, the way in which the job is conducted and undertaken on a daily basis, is as important as a job description. The key to successful job design is to provide a match between job design, individual employee abilities and preferences, and organizational demands on the particular job position. A manager or executive who optimizes resources will be able to make this match successfully in most situations.

Significant Responsibility

The level of responsibility an employee holds is determined by job content and design and is closely aligned with the authority held in a particular position. The responsibility for making decisions, prioritizing various aspects of the job, and balancing the work load is inherent in almost every job in a health care organization.

Although the majority of responsibilities held by the employee in a particular job position are spelled out in the job description, most organizations expect employees to take on additional responsibilities that are not specified in the job description but that must be undertaken occasionally. These responsibilities are referred to as "significant contribution" and should also be delineated for the employee and understood fully.

Some employees desire to make more significant contributions to their jobs than do other employees. An example is a supervisor who desires to take on myriad professional responsibilities—supervisory responsibilities, technical responsibilities, and professional management responsibilities. Other employees are content merely to perform one routinized scheme of activities, with little change or additional responsibilities from day to day. In either case, an employee's significant contribution to the organization should be evaluated along with the job standards specified in the job description because all are part of the organization's expectations. Section III of the value-driven performance evaluation plan in appendix B presents an evaluation form for recording employee performance that is clearly significant and/or above and beyond the call of duty.

Communication

Communication on a job is an important aspect of leadership, starting in the executive suite and working down to the lower echelons of first-line management. A successful health care manager must be able to understand that communication is the key to understanding employees.

Health care managers must be flexible in terms of the type of communication they provide, the style in which that communication is delivered, and, perhaps most important, the listening skills and perceptual abilities they demonstrate in their interaction with employees on a daily basis. Employees who feel as though they are never "heard," or never "understood," will quickly become dissatisfied. These individuals are chronically not allowed to venture their opinions, and, in many cases, provide meaningless insight into the way that a particular work objective can be achieved or a project undertaken. Furthermore, the lack of attention given to their particular work input is also detrimental to their personal self-esteem and perceived value to the organization.

As has already been demonstrated, a part of any job design and job description should be the means for good communication between the individual and the supervising manager or executive. Furthermore, individuality and a respect for the dignity of each individual should be taken into account. In other words, each employee is different, and thus has a different level of interest in communicating with his or her manager. Managers must understand the "independence" factor, that is, the degree of attention that needs to be given to each employee and the level of communication to be undertaken between each employee and the manager in the interest of performing at an optimum level.

Negative Consequences

Each job in a health care organization carries a certain potential for negative consequences for poor performance. Going back to the universal example of the plow horse, these consequences represent the "stick" attendant to the motivation of each job. Negative motivation is intrinsic to every job. In health care, dire consequences are part of the negative consequences of a job. Dire consequences, or negative outcomes, can be attributed to the pharmacist who delivers a prescription in the wrong quantity or composition, a hospital security guard who wrongfully hassles a relative visiting a seriously ill customer/patient, or a housekeeper who leaves the floor of a high-traffic ward wet, making it dangerous for patients and for medical personnel hurrying on their rounds and appointed duties.

The negative consequences of every given job should be portrayed accurately and adequately to each employee at the outset as part of the orientation process. These consequences should then be reinforced through counseling, as appropriate throughout a grading period, and underscored tangibly during the performance evaluation discussion. Health care is unique in that the negative consequences of a job performed poorly can spell the difference between good health and bad health, even life and death. It is therefore essential for the manager to communicate the potential consequences of poor performance for each particular job position, leading up to and including suspension and termination for employees who chronically reap negative outcomes to their assigned responsibilities.

Work Climate

Another job-related motivator is work climate, that is, the environmental and psychological factors that create a productive work environment. For example, does the work climate have ample lighting, desk space, and noise control? Does the work climate encourage open communication and autonomy of responsibilities, or do employees rely on a supervisor for hour-by-hour instruction and guidance?

The work climate, then, is the way in which work is undertaken, supervised, and judged as positive or negative. The work climate can also connote the "personality" of a particular department or organization. Some work climates generate a high degree of stress, as do many health care organizations; this stress can be augmented by the geographic location of a facility. For example, the work climate in the emergency room of a major municipal hospital in New York City is bound to be frenzied and stressful, because that organization operates as a public trust to individuals in a very turbulent environment. The work climate in a residential home for the aging in a rural section of Alabama might be less frenzied, yet have the same attendant responsibilities of high care and optimum performance. The difference between the two is the pace of work and the level of high-pressure activity inherent in everyday responsibilities, both of which are obviously heightened by the type of job performed and its role in the organization.

Some people are highly motivated by the "action" attending a large municipal organization; others enjoy the relatively slow pace of a rural facility. There is a distinct link between the work climate within which a certain job operates, the attributes an individual needs to successfully undertake that job, and the responsibilities of the job itself. Once again, given the individual orientation of the employee, the progressive health care manager must ensure a match between the individual's desire for an appropriate work climate, and realistic expectations contained within the job, organization, and environment at hand.

Whenever a manager discusses a new position with an employee or applicant, he or she must describe the level of stress in a given job. Mismatching a high-stress position to an employee with a low stress tolerance paves the way for a soon-to-be-open position.

The manager must also adequately address levels of stress for existing employees. Most health care employees enjoy (or can tolerate) the quick pace of action and the high degree of pressure within their job. Otherwise, they would not last within the health care environment for very long. However, each job has a certain level of stress, which must be recognized and controlled if it is to be a positive and not a negative motivator over the long haul.

Job Advancement and Enhancement

Some health care workers aspire to become CEOs or top administrators in a health care organization. Others are content to retain their current role, possible adding new responsibilities periodically.

For employees who aspire to a top-level position in the health care field, advancement is a motivator that becomes an important part of job design. The avenues by which an individual can advance to the upper tiers of management must be assessed and presented to the employee, along with a strategy for attaining these career goals.

Employees who simply want their jobs enhanced with new responsibilities from time to time must determine with their managers how this can be done. For example, the employee might learn to use a different piece of equipment, perform more projects within a given realm of activity, or learn to use time and monetary resources more efficiently.

Without job advancement and enhancement opportunities, individual motivation is not optimized, and employee contributions to the organization's objectives are not met fully.

☐ Jointly Established Motivators

Motivators established jointly by the individual and the organization (that is, its management team and the job description) include the following:

- *Appreciation techniques:* Methods by which the organization and its managers show their gratitude to the employee for work output and dedication to high-quality health care service
- *Expectations/outcomes:* Short- and mid-range goals established between the employee and managers to step up challenges and level of accomplishment
- *Future objectives:* Long-term plans and goals in which the employee will participate and gain technical knowledge and ongoing professional development as an integral member of the work group
- *Mutual benefit:* Establishment of goals and objectives that result in positive action, which provides clear benefits to the organization, respective management members, and the employee
- *Pride:* Groupwide interpersonal investment in the workplace, as reflected in a commitment to group goal attainment and a feeling of self-fulfillment from group achievement
- *Professional development:* Opportunities identified and facilitated by management for the employee to increase job-related knowledge, technical acumen, and business prowess
- *Work ethic:* Application of effort demanded by management from the employee on a daily basis, as well as employee dedication, desire for success, and determination to meet established goals
- *Work norms:* Daily pattern of work activity regulated and administered by managers in the interest of maximizing workplace action and optimizing employee comfort and productivity
- *Workplace interaction:* Relative harmony within a given working environment, marked by a spirit of cooperation and cohesiveness

To provide some examples of jointly established motivators, some appreciation techniques might include raises, promotions, or other incentives permitted by the budget. Demonstration of appreciation is a jointly established motivator because the individual employee has the responsibility to state during a performance review what he or she wants from the job; as a group, employees should tell the organization what they desire as motivation to work fruitfully over a long term.

Pride, work ethic, and work norms are interrelated motivators. The individual who takes significant pride in his or her job helps to bring about a good group work ethic within the department, which establishes a cultural norm of hard work, perseverance, and dedication to duty throughout the organization. The strong presence of these three motivators must start with the exemplary conduct provided by the top executive, filter down through the organization, and be embraced by all members of the organization.

☐ Practical Applications

The culture of an organization should encourage the use of motivators to inspire peak performance and gain maximum commitment from every employee. When every individual wants to maximize performance and commitment to corporate standards of conduct, the organization usually has a harmonious workplace, in that everyone is working toward the same objective. As the old adage goes, "the person rowing the boat seldom has time to rock it." With this in mind, an organization that provides a strong sense of corporate direction and ethical standards in the workplace—and encourages employees to participate in the establishment of organizational goals—will be successful in the long run and provide its patient/customer community with high- quality health care.

The following practical applications may serve to examine the extent to which employee motivators are present in your organization or department.

1. Review all of the motivators in the chapter and determine how they affect your personal performance.
2. Determine which organizational motivators are most apparent in your organization, as well as which are most lacking.
3. Conduct a review of the motivational factors as they relate to your reporting staff.
4. If you are an executive, determine how the motivational factors affect your board and which ones are most powerful to their interaction with your organizational management.
5. Use the definitions of motivators in appendix C with your staff as a team development exercise.
6. Supplement the list of motivators by adding your own specific dynamics of motivation to the list.

7. Objectively determine which motivators are most important to your peers and colleagues in management.
8. Assess which *category* of motivators is most important to you.
9. Assess which motivators are *not* important and why.
10. Which motivator would be most effective in your boss's management strategy? Use this as a premise in your next discussion with him or her.

Chapter 5

Management of Conflict, Change, and Cultural Diversity

The health care manager in a progressive organization must do more than employ a set of motivators and shared values to lead staff effectively toward desired goals. The manager must also manage the dynamics of conflict, change, and cultural differences to maximize staff performance. This chapter examines these dynamics, their interaction, and their effective management through strategies that enable the reader to garner positive outcomes whenever possible.

Conflict in the health care workplace can be a most damaging force. When employees find a source of conflict and, in their collective perception, the manager does not resolve it quickly, resolutely, and clearly, the conflict can fester and hamper productivity and quality of care. Conflict in the workplace can be found in many sources—interpersonal clashes, differing agendas, divided loyalties, interdepartmental agendas and objectives. In any case, unless the health care manager addresses the source of conflict and resolves the negative aspects, a problem can accelerate over time.

Change is an ever-present dynamic that exists at every level of a health care organization. Change is threatening to many health care employees and represents a variation to the status quo and the potential for prohibiting goal accomplishment and consequently the employees' feeling of accomplishment and achievement. Change takes many forms in the health care workplace—work direction, work norms, and methods of obtaining results, for example. The very nature of the profession and the business dynamics involved in the modern health care setting all incorporate a certain amount of change. The manager who can present change openly and positively to the staff has a distinct advantage not only in surviving, but thriving in a health care organization.

Pluralism in the health care workplace mandates that the manager be sensitive to the dynamics of cultural diversity as well, for example, the various ethnic groups that comprise most health care work forces. Another form of cultural diversity is the corporate culture established by the leadership of a progressive health care organization and administered and reinforced by its line management. Finally, certain subcultures exist within a health care organization. For example, nurses seem to breed a culture of their own; lab technicians, another. Broadly defined, a *culture* is any group that shares common goals and norms within a health care workplace based on ethnic, demographic, or technical communality.

Conflict, change, and cultural diversity are ever-present variables in the work life of any health care manager, as the rest of this chapter demonstrates.

□ Managing Conflict

Conflict can exist within the health care organization on many different planes. The first key to resolving conflict within a work group is to identify its cause.

Causes of Conflict

Within a health care organization several types of conflict are common:

1. *Interdepartmental conflict:* Interdepartmental conflict arises between the differing goals and objectives of two or more departments or work groups within a department. Although various work groups within an organization are all motivated toward service provision, each has its own set of goals and objectives and work norms in accomplishing the results desired throughout the work cycle. As such, interdepartmental conflict can exist between two departments with varying agendas, goals, and ways of accomplishing those goals.
2. *Political conflict:* Political conflict can also occur within an organization, particularly at levels where critical decisions are made and organizational agendas are established. Politics is fundamentally the process of management by a group of individuals. Because of differences in personality, objectives, and communication styles, it is only natural that in any organization—health care or otherwise—certain political conflicts might occur. More pragmatically, however, differing agendas and priorities can cause conflict not only in terms of policy interpretation, but also relative to basic goals and objectives of the organization and the manner in which those objectives are reached.
3. *Cultural conflict:* Cultural conflict can exist within an organization on several levels. The most apparent is conflict based on ethnic or

demographic preference. Although this is the most apparent type of cultural conflict, it is also the least common due to the heightened awareness and workers' rights and equal opportunity legislation. Nonetheless, cultural conflict is potentially the most divisive type of conflict, in that it is founded on hatred and fear. This type of conflict is easily recognized and remedied by swift corrective action, discussed later in this section.

4. *Organization versus department conflict:* Organization versus department conflict occurs when a certain department considers itself to be more important than the goals and objectives of the organization, or the organization itself. Frequently ascribed to physician groups, this dilemma can extend to virtually any type of organizational entity. The inherent danger in this type of conflict is that any department, or departments, allowed to consider itself more important than the organization will become elitist in nature and begin to see other departments as inferior. Because a health care organization is made up of divergent services that are highly technical in nature and equally important in the provision of care to the customer/patient, it is easy to see how this type of conflict is fundamentally harmful to the organization. Moreover, no organization can truly achieve a sense of unity and strength if each of its segments considers itself most important.

5. *Individual versus work group conflict:* Within a specific department, a certain individual might consider himself or herself more important than the entire department. This is usually called the "superstar complex," meaning that the individual feels superior to the rest of the work team. This complex causes conflict from several different angles. First, this individual might cause animosity within the work group as individuals come to resent this stance as manifested in their communication style and attitude. Second, this "superstar" might argue continually or interrupt certain work dynamics if he or she considers the work directive personally insulting. Third—without delving too much into the psychological aspects—this individual is often insecure and thus will need a lot of attention and esteem from the manager, which will take away valuable time and energy from the rest of the work group, in turn creating yet another source of resentment.

6. *Racial/sexual conflict:* Aspects of racial and sexual conflict within the work group legally are defined as discrimination or harassment. Despite a great deal of attention and awareness within the American workplace relative to these dynamics, unfortunately their perils still exist. In that a health care setting is representative of the community and provides a basic human service, racism and sexism can be devastating.

7. *Change-related conflict:* Change-related conflict is prevalent in the health care setting almost daily. Because of the sweeping changes in the

health care field itself, the progressive health care organization must be flexible and readily adaptable in terms of type of services offered, methods of service provision, and other business dynamics. Change can also exist relative to technological approaches and basic operational facets of the workplace. Change must be managed successfully, as will be discussed in the next section, but more important, any conflict arising because of change should be dealt with proactively.

Conflict within the workplace, no matter what its nature, must be dealt with as clearly, quickly, resolutely, and fairly as possible. Although theoretically these dynamics sound very reasonable and act as an ideal solution to conflict, in practice they become very difficult. Health care managers wrestle with the problem of conflict and approach it in several different ways; nevertheless, it is difficult to deal with conflict objectively.

Why Conflict Is Difficult to Deal With

It is difficult for managers to deal with conflict because it produces six by-products that affect both manager and work group. First, conflict becomes very taxing on the manager who must spend valuable time away from key tasks trying to resolve the conflict.

Second, conflict causes a severe acrimony within the work group. The source of conflict is exacerbated when various parties discuss and offer their viewpoints and solutions. In consulting to large health care organizations, the author has experienced many situations where a conflict remained unresolved for a long time. It became a bigger source of contention in the department, to the point of becoming a divisive element among department members. The result was, in effect, two different departments, complete with two different agendas, work norms, and cultures.

A third by-product of conflict is avoidance. Department members will use the conflict as an excuse to avoid a particular issue—which might be the very issue that generated the conflict. Even more damaging, the individuals involved in the conflict might avoid each other, which creates factionalism within the work group, prohibits open and sound communication, and results in lost productivity and unacceptable quality. This stifles their opportunity to develop and grow and to prosper.

A fourth by-product is ignorance, which, for purposes of this discussion can have two implications. Individuals who ignore a situation not only avoid addressing the problem but refuse to enlighten themselves about the situation or the people involved. This makes it impossible to apply education and technical knowledge properly if people deliberately ignore key situations or the insights of a particular group of team members in a work unit.

Furthermore, if given the opportunity, people will pretend that the situation does not exist. That is, the dynamics of the situation, as well as the individuals involved, are not deemed pertinent to their particular interests.

A fifth by-product of conflict is that the conflict becomes an alibi for poor work performance—"We can't do this because you know how so and so is" or "We can't do this because you know what happened last time." In the first statement, worker X is using worker Y as scapegoat for worker X's poor performance. In the latter statement, the worker is citing a past work experience as an excuse not to perform at all. In both cases, an objective is jeopardized that could have been attained had the source of conflict been addressed concisely and constructively in the first place.

Finally, if allowed to fester and grow, a source of conflict can affect a work group's morale over time. In the first place, the work group leader is seen as incompetent—"Well, what do you expect, he/she wasn't able to handle _____"—and as a result, confidence in his or her leadership will be shaken. In the second place, confidence in the work group's ability to act together progressively as a unit to solve its problems will be eroded. Collectively, the work group will distrust its ability to provide the top-quality services that are the organization's mission.

Dealing with Group Conflict

To deal with conflict constructively, the health care manager must use a strategy that is comprehensive enough to encompass all types of conflict. The first step toward resolution is communication; the manager must seek out from all parties concerned the basic elements of the conflict, potential solutions, and a time line for resolution. This is accomplished by asking questions, not by making assumptions about the source of the conflict, the reasons for the conflict, or how various individuals will respond. The manger should ask:

1. What are the major problems?
2. Why does this conflict exist?
3. How is this conflict affecting us?
4. What solutions do you see for the conflict?
5. How quickly should we address some of these conflicts?
6. What would you do if you were in my position?

By asking these questions and listening closely to the answers, the manager collects data that identify all aspects of conflict source as well as potential solutions. Furthermore, a progressive communication strategy is needed to solve the conflict with clarity, completeness, compassion, and closure.

The next step is for the manager to garner resources needed to resolve the conflict. This could be as simple as securing a conference room for a group discussion or as complex as securing physical or additional financial resources.

For example, assume that a food-service unit in a rural hospital has been directed by the administration to change its menu for inpatient services. The reason for this change is unclear to many of the food-service personnel, a work group divided between two ethnic lines and perceived throughout the facility as being purely a support group. The food-service manager in appraising the situation anticipates a conflict due to the change in work direction. The conflict is also expected to be compounded by the cultural diversity of the work group; the manager knows that morale is low because the group perceives itself to be held in low esteem by the organization.

In applying the first step of the resolution strategy to this situation— communication—the manager of the food-service department would have the entire group meet on company time at a time convenient for everyone in the department. A common mistake managers make is to try to solve conflict past working hours; this sends an implicit message to the parties that the conflict is either not important or is something that must be done in addition to the regular work duties. Recall that conflict is a distinct threat to the conduct of regular work activities and thus must be implicitly recognized as such. In working with this initial meeting group, the food-service manager will ask the questions enumerated in the preceding paragraphs. The desired outcome is first to diffuse the perception of conflict in the group; that is, to let individuals vent their anxiety about changing the work direction. After garnering appropriate suggestions from the group, the food-service manager should also endeavor to establish the following important points.

First, the manager should express to the group the need to work together from a good-business standpoint. Despite past differences or cultural differences, the work group will be successful only to the extent that the individuals involved are successful. That is, no one will win unless everyone wins.

With this thought in mind, the manager should move to the second step in the resolution effort—gathering resources for a solution. He or she should try to establish some key objectives that can be achieved within an established time frame. For example, in this case the food-service manager might establish a new menu and delivery system that can be implemented for inpatient services within a two-month time limit. The manager might then work from the general to the specific, that is, ask for specific ideas from the work group on how to accomplish each key objective. Any enthusiasm shown for a particular idea from a group member should then turn into a "contribution objective." This means that the objective based on the suggested idea becomes a group goal. This goal should be incorporated into the performance appraisal cycle and have an attendant reward attached to it. By establishing finite goals, the manager establishes "watermarks" for progress and success in the group process.

Dealing with Conflict Caused by One Individual

The example in the previous section illustrates a group process toward conflict resolution. Another strategy might be used in dealing with conflict caused by one individual. Recall from an earlier discussion the conflict caused by the "superstar" complex. In this situation, the manager must use a different communication strategy, which may be called the *E-formula*. This formula consists of the following components:

- Evidence: Illustrating negative impact on poor performance
- Example: Demonstrating clearly the specific performance problems
- Effect: Operating on the individual's work role and the entire work unit
- Exemplar: Representing model behavior and desired actions in the work role
- Education: Providing individual guidance on how to improve performance

First, *evidence* must be collected to show the negative effect of the individual's actions on his or her performance, such as dereliction of duty. The evidence should be quantified as much as possible—that is, losses in terms of a percentage, number, or amount of time or money. Evidence that cannot be quantified and hence is less clearly defined should also be exposed, such as any emotionalism or resentment that precludes success in the workplace.

Second, the manager must present to the individual involved in the conflict a set of specific *examples* that have contributed to conflict in the workplace. This includes any clear instances of performance below the standard required by the manager or that varied in scope and effectiveness from the goals established. These examples should be easily recognized by the employee so as to minimize the opportunity for debate or contention during a one-on-one counseling session. All examples should be tied to performance, and as many examples as are appropriate should be discussed. *Note:* The use of one or two clearly defined and readily recognizable examples is just as effective as six or seven obscure examples.

Next, the manager should demonstrate clearly what *effect* the employee's behavior is having on colleagues or on the entire work process. This demonstration includes any effects on productivity as well as on the morale of specific employees or the entire work group. Furthermore, the manager should try to personalize the effect on the employee; for example, show how the problematic behavior is affecting his or her performance, goal accomplishment, and morale. The manager then should emphasize that this behavior will not be tolerated and delineate the specific negative consequences that might occur if the employee fails to modify the behavior and the approach to work.

At this juncture, the manager should elicit from the employee the (1) reasons why he or she is creating the conflict, (2) other evidence the employee feels might be pertinent to the discussion, and (3) explanation of the conflict's effect on the employee from his or her own viewpoint. This three-prong opportunity ensures that the discussion is comprehensive and allows the employee to begin to participate in the more positive aspects of the discussion still to come.

The fourth component of the E-formula, *exemplar*, depicts the level of excellence to which the manager expects the employee to aspire. With the employee's assistance, the manager establishes what the desired performance is, that is, outcomes and specific behaviors. This not only serves to correct the conflict caused by the employee, it sets a standard for what must be accomplished and how.

It is imperative for the employee to understand how the job must be done and how he or she can aspire to the standards of the exemplar. The manager may ask the employee for suggestions on how the desired performance can be attained, and specifically to address ways in which the manager might assist the employee in reaching goals and behavioral objectives.

The final component of the E-formula is *education*. The manager must apprise the employee on at least four aspects of his or her future behavior:

1. The employee's conflict-causing behavior will not be tolerated under any circumstances.
2. The manager, by virtue of this conversation and willingness to discuss the issues at any time with the employee on an individual basis, stands ready to assist the employee to attain the desired performance.
3. The manager will encourage the employee to seek out any assistance that will contribute to doing a better job and accomplishing objectives in a manner that is satisfying to all involved.
4. The manager must express confidence in the employee's ability to attain the desired results and to act as a viable, progressive entity to the job.

In health care organizations, "turfdom" might exist between groups, and antipathy might exist among individuals. In both approaches to conflict resolution—group and individual—the manager must underline the fact that the mission and objectives of the organization are paramount to any individual or group concerns. By using these two strategies, conflict can be resolved proactively and quickly so that performance is redirected toward progressive goals. In all cases, communication is the key, as is the guided participation of the parties involved.

☐ Managing Change

Managing change in the health care environment is a complex process in that change is almost a daily occurrence throughout the workplace, where every day is an adventure. However, some clear elements of change can be recognized, and a systematic formula can be applied in presenting change toward a positive and progressive end.

Change exists in the health care workplace for a number of reasons. First, the highly technical nature of this field creates constant flux as new technological advances take hold and new systems are installed.

Second, the customer/patient base is diverse in scope and is also constantly changing. Witness such dynamics as the aging population and the increased activity of those enjoying their golden years in an active life-style. This phenomenon mandates an entire range of service provision to senior citizens. Also, new maladies afflict the health care patient population, from the more widely recognized illnesses such as AIDS to the less apparent ones such as addiction to gambling. These contemporary afflictions mandate a change in services and flexibility of approach from all health care professionals.

Third, the health care worker and the requirements of his or her daily activities are undergoing a drastic change. Increased public scrutiny and more regulation of service delivery have mandated a series of changes over the past 10 years that have been dramatic and swift.

Common Mistakes in Addressing Change

In dealing with change, a manager can make four major mistakes to the detriment of his or her own effectiveness, as well as to that of the assigned staff. First, the manager can deny the existence of change, whether to a specific change that is affecting the department or to a change throughout the organization. In doing so, the manager exposes himself or herself to staff charges of mendaciousness or insensitivity toward the particular element of change. Furthermore, such denial compromises a fundamental link of integrity between the manager and the employee, diminishing the faith that employees have in the manager to react positively to change and to maintain the progressive action of the work group.

The second major mistake a manager can make is to ignore any impending change or any aspects of change. This can take the form of not addressing a particular element of change, not communicating to the employees the forthcoming change in a workplace, or perhaps not publicly recognizing a need to change or a new dynamic to the workplace. This kind of managerial obliviousness inadvertently declares a leader as ignorant of trends in his or her technical area of management responsibilities. Consequently, the employee's faith in the manager's intelligence, empathy, and technical skills is jeopardized. Furthermore, the employees might take it upon themselves to try to react to change, thus usurping the leadership of their work group. All of these are obviously negative consequences, all rooted in managerial ignorance and failure to respond effectively to change, or, simply put, to ignore the need to change.

A third mistake is made when the manager alters, embellishes, or slants the impending change, that is, endeavors to put a "different light" on the change dynamic. This different light might be fundamentally untrue, inappropriate, or simply a misstatement of the facts. In any case, it will be perceived as being dishonest by the employees and once again compromise the allegiance between the employees and the manager.

Consider the example of a personnel manager who must implement a new job evaluation system. If the personnel manager, in discussing the new program with the staff, overstates the positive nature of the job evaluation system, underestimates the amount of work involved to make the change, and omits key factors of implementation the staff will be expected to perform, not only is the allegiance of the staff diminished but, more important, their performance level suffers. Obviously, the breach of integrity and the other value-driven factors can result in a morale problem that will directly affect performance in this case. Not only will it be more difficult to complete the implementation of the job evaluation system, but the system may be a source of conflict in the long run in this particular department.

Finally, the health care manager who tries to contend with or fight change risks the negative consequences. A manager's resistance to change, which is often compounded by a contagious resistance from within the rest of the work group, can have a pejorative effect on the individual employee, the department, and in many cases the entire organization. A department perceived as being resistant to change is seen as being reactive and ineffective. A leader who is resistant to change is perceived as being behind the times.

A manager who is resistant to change is seen as lacking loyalty, expertise, commitment to the organization, and leadership skills. This type of manager will often pose as a victim of change, or perhaps a "martyr" of change. A victim of change contends so strongly that change will be negative that he or she ultimately will make no changes within the work group or to the way work is performed (not even necessary changes).

A martyr of change will undertake the change but complain assiduously about it to the point that the organization and the staff will wish the change never occurred and come to dread any change that must be made within the organization.

With all four reactions to change, the negative common denominator is that change will not be done in a proactive fashion, thus presenting the liability that the change will not be done effectively and efficiently. Furthermore, poor reaction to change, if it permeates a health care organization, will shift the organization's progressive direction to a regressive one. Finally, the cultural norm throughout the organization will be one that discounts change as a vital necessity and thus misses opportunities to service its customer/patient base and to keep pace with the health care community.

Strategies for Managing Change

Two strategies must be used in presenting change and garnering support for undertaking a change in the way work is performed. The first strategy is a *presentation strategy,* the objective of which is to present the need for the change, the way in which the change will benefit all parties involved, and, finally, the entire organization. The second strategy is an *implementation strategy,* which is needed to effect action relative to the change and define specific roles for performance and for undertaking the change.

By applying these two strategies, the manager can objectively and systematically address the ever-present dynamics of change on a regular basis. In this way, change now becomes not a detriment to motivation and productivity but a measurable asset in attaining productivity and ensuring progress in the health care workplace.

The Presentation Strategy

Presentation of a change should be done as a group process if a group will be involved in implementing the change, or as an individual process if the change will affect only one individual or one work role. The first step of the presentation strategy is to openly present the objective of the change. The critical aspect many health care managers and executives overlook in implementing change is to stress how the change will improve the status quo of the organization, including the way the individual does a particular job. If there is no improvement to the current situation, it is indeed a tough "sell" for the manager to present change. Change just for change's sake is usually resented by employees and seen as a worthless exercise. In addition, organizational morale will suffer. However, if an organization is always changing to upgrade its services, the change is usually more easily acceptable, acknowledged, and embraced by all sectors of the organization.

In this first step of the presentation strategy, the manager should ask the employees to visualize specifically the new dimensions of the change. For example, if a security force at a large metropolitan hospital is asked to change the way it conducts rounds during the night shift, the visualization technique would be used to ask patrolling security officers to visualize what the new rounds and physical presence of the guards at key locations might "look like" to potential intruders. As another example, a computer operator might be asked how much easier the job would be if a new program was put into place, in effect to visualize what the job would "look like." In undertaking this exercise, the manager accomplishes two objectives: first, presentation of a positive, clear vision of why the change will bring about an improvement, and second, the benefit of eliciting from the employee an idealized contribution to the vision, which in turn invites the employee to share the vision. Now the change and the reasons for it become an integral part of the employee's work life and work objectives. Hopefully, this will also encourage a certain amount of employee enthusiasm for the change.

In the second step of the presentation strategy, it is important for the manager to explain to employees the rationale for why a change is taking place. In the countless attitude surveys conducted by the author, the only time a change is resented by employees is when they have not been told why the change is taking place. Hence, it is recommended that the employee be given insight by the manager as to why a change is taking place—in essence, the rationalization and reasoning process for the change. Failure to do so runs the risk of insulting the employee's intelligence and belies his or her expertise about the organization and the job. Furthermore, the change hints of "their" change as opposed to "our" change, that is, it becomes more of a directive than a collective, participative project. Employees might not necessarily agree with the rationale for the change, but at least they are not precluded from understanding and recognizing the manager's rationale for making the change. Acceptance and understanding are two different elements. Whereas the employees might not accept the manager's rationale, at least by understanding it their own self-esteem and self-worth regarding technical expertise is not ignored. Furthermore, an astute health care manager will ask employees for ways in which this change might assist them and their work roles. In essence, the rationale is expanded to include not only the organizational and managerial viewpoint, but the employees' viewpoint as well.

The third step is for the manager to explain the short-term implementation strategy and the long-term benefits the change will incur. In this step, the manager should balance the increases in effectiveness and quality resulting from the long-term change with the inefficiencies and decreases in quantity of work resulting from the short-term change. Any type of change requires an increase of effort and time on the part of the staff, which might inconvenience their work norms as well as infringe on their time and ability to maintain high-quality output. However, the long-term effect will be greater productivity and efficiency and an increase in quality. In fact, if this long-term effect is not in the offing relative to the change dynamic, the change should not occur. In presenting the short- and long-term strategies, dealing with them explicitly and frankly, the manager establishes a certain level of empathy with the employees and pledges their participation in the change process.

Finally, the presentation strategy should communicate the effect of the change on the individual employee as well as the department and the organization as a whole. For example, to return to the case of the food-service department earlier in this chapter, the manager might stress the creative opportunities for the employees to participate in the new food-service project, the efficiency that the department will now have, and the additional services that will be provided to the organization. Or, to consider once again the case of the personnel administrator in the job evaluation program, the administrator might communicate the efficiencies brought to each job and the overall improvements in organizational morale, which will be gained through a clear job evaluation system. All three levels—the individual, department, and organization—should be presented to give the employee a full perspective of the need for change, its benefits, and its overall contribution to the organizational and individual welfare of the health care institution.

The Implementation Strategy

The presentation strategy must be augmented with the implementation strategy. Beyond explaining to staff the relevance of the change to the big picture, and beyond reinforcing the common purpose across the department—all serving to demystify the change—the manager must now de-personalize the change by using an implementation strategy that stresses the mutual benefit and a "win-win-win" approach.

To attain this objective, the manager must ask the employees the following key questions:

- What are the major reasons for this change?
- Why is this change important?
- How does this change affect you and your job?
- How can we decrease the negative factors of this change?
- What role(s) do you want to play in this change situation?
- What benefits will this change provide to the organization?

- How will this change benefit you and your work role?
- What long-term benefits will this change provide to the organization?
- What additional resources do you need to undergo this process?
- What can I do to make this process more efficient and effective for you?

By asking these questions, the manager will discover what each employee can contribute to the project and get a fuller perspective for implementing the needed change. The manager might also discover a "better way" of implementing the change and garner the depth of each employee's expertise in the range of change for each work role. This not only allows each employee to participate actively, it provides some fruitful results in planning the change.

The manager–employee dialogue must be augmented by assurances of the mutual benefits to all parties involved. These include the benefits of the change to the organization, how those benefits will enhance the employee's stability and security in the organizational work force, and how the change will benefit the department in terms of efficiency and effectiveness. In underscoring this point, the manager ensures that the employees realize that the change not only will affect everyone but will benefit everyone in the long run.

☐ Managing Cultural Diversity

As emphasized throughout this book, a progressive health care organization embraces a value-driven approach toward managing people in a realistic manner. This includes the implementation of an organizational culture that utilizes the strategies and performance values delineated throughout this text. Nevertheless, various subcultures exist in any health care workplace, and various cultural issues arising from ethnic, gender-based, and other demographic factors can be destructive if not managed properly.

The Risks of Improper Management

The health care manager who allows cultural conflict to occur runs several risks. First and most apparent is the legal issue of liability incurred. Under Title VII, discrimination in the workplace based on sex, ethnic or racial heritage, or certain other protected categories can have drastic repercussions to both the manager and the organization. Additionally, an organization found to be illegally biased will suffer negative word-of-mouth publicity throughout the community.

Second, organizational values are subverted by cultural differences within the workplace. Any organization experiencing cultural conflict of any kind cannot have a true value-driven system of management. This absence of values might be reflected not only in productivity but in quality of service to the customer/patient. It will also disengender team performance and strong organizational galvanization.

Third, with increasing media attention to health care, any organizational problems stemming from cultural differences will be well publicized and will negatively affect the health care organization's business affairs, including the dynamics of ethnic rivalries and union factionalism.

As for individual employees, cultural conflict between two groups within a department can cause a variety of problems. For example, communication might suffer as people "forget" to share information, or different factions might refuse to work cooperatively, thus endangering goal attainment. Furthermore, certain emotional responses might prompt open confrontation. Covert discrimination might affect promotions and inclusion in key work activities or in pertinent job assignments. The end result in all these instances is detriment to health care provision.

Management Techniques

Indicators of potential cultural conflict include the following:

- Stereotyping
- Ethnic jokes and slurs
- Discourse communicating a "they/us" or "those people" mentality
- Passive aggressiveness (such as not following up on requests after agreeing to take action)
- Lack of communication altogether
- Nonverbal indicators (such as folded arms or other body language expressing displeasure)

A manager must use several techniques to quash cultural conflict. First, overt discrimination must be dealt with quickly and openly. Therefore, it is imperative for the manager to confront these situations, preferably with the assistance of a capable human resources executive. A third party ensures objectivity and lends to the process professional expertise.

Second, the chain of command must be adhered to. The manager's superior should act as a mentor in this area, meaning that this executive should take a vital role in resolving cultural conflict in the organization and in any reporting department. Once again, a human resources specialist is key, but the additional expertise of a manager experienced in this area adds to the equation in a positive way. The manager should address cultural differences through performance evaluations and other organizational mechanisms. Criteria and standards as set forth in this book can be incorporated not only into the performance evaluation strategies but into new employee orientations and other aspects of the employee's work life.

Third, in dealing with cultural differences, as with other types of conflict in the health care workplace, the manager must utilize certain keys, the first of which is communication. Managers should look for any signs of cultural conflict (see above indicators), listen, and communicate effectively that cultural conflict—whether of the corporate culture or ethnic or gender-based culture—will not be tolerated. This should be done openly and equitably, starting with each employee's or supervisor's first day of employment.

Another key is to make sure that all employees understand that they are part of the big picture, meaning they have to work together, communicate effectively, and inform the manager of any problems they might have. Inherent in this is a need for the manager to work with employees at their own comfort level, that is, asking employees key questions; making sure that feedback is kept confidential not just during the annual performance evaluation, but throughout the work cycle; and ensuring that shy, reticent employees are given the same opportunity to give feedback as the more outspoken employees are.

No radical groups should be allowed to exist in the organization. This includes groups who perceive themselves as being elitist or groups consisting of individuals who find a common interest in inhibiting progressive performance. Direct confrontation, clear communication, and conflict resolution are together the best solution to disarming such groups.

Because of the serious nature of cultural conflict, progressive discipline must be applied when warranted. Employees should first be given verbal warnings, then written warnings, and finally probationary notices if their negative conduct continues. Therefore, good documentation is mandatory; the manager must keep records of specific dates, actions taken, and clear-cut evidence and examples of delinquent performance and negative behavior that interfere with employees' equal opportunity to perform their jobs optimally. This progressive discipline cycle must be reinforced by the facility's leadership, administered by all levels of management, and communicated to all employees. It must be the norm and not the exception.

Finally, in hiring practices, utilizing the questions or "cues" in appendix A will give a progressive health care organization an edge in attracting employees who will not create or foster cultural conflict in the organization, and specifically in their area of job responsibility.

☐ Practical Applications

In light of the turbulence in the U.S. business environment, and specifically in the health care business environment, any type of internal conflict can threaten the stability of the entire organization. It is the responsibility of every manager—not just the CEO—to manage conflict ardently and successfully, whether that conflict is spawned by change, cultural differences, or other individual or group behaviors.

Conflict allowed to linger can destroy morale, productivity, and overall quality of health care provision. Most of all, it can threaten the life of a patient/customer as well as the organization itself. When conflict is addressed quickly, resolutely, and fairly, a very important message is sent to all employees: "Our organization does not merely pay lip service to the maximization of employee abilities and contributions; rather, it is committed to making employee development a way of life." As a result, morale is increased, productivity is increased, and all members of the organization embrace the health care organization as a viable, progressive, and exemplary facility in which to practice their profession.

The following applications may serve as a starting place for honing your ability to manage conflict, change, and cultural diversity:

1. Review the action strategies delineated in this chapter with all subordinate supervisors and team leaders.
2. Incorporate all of these strategies into your training and development programs that deal with supervisory techniques.
3. Monitor your staff for any indicators of conflict, change, or problems stemming from cultural diversity, based on the criteria listed in the text.
4. Use the E-formula in the next conflict management situation you encounter.
5. Use the dynamics of change management in the next situation of this kind that you encounter.
6. Use the text material on cultural conflict to deal quickly and resolutely with any problems in this area.
7. Utilize all of the material in this section when undertaking the responsibilities of managing a new department or set of responsibilities, because all of these dynamics are present in those "turnaround" and "takeover" situations.
8. Encourage staff participation in all change situations, using the strategies outlined in the text.
9. Recognize that all three dynamics—change, conflict, and cultural diversity—can work integrally as well as separately, so that in some cases a combination of strategies might be needed.
10. Use this material proactively, not just reactively.

Chapter 6

Critical Line Management Strategies

In practicing their trade in a turbulent, ever-changing environment, health care managers are constantly challenged by a wide array of emergent issues that affect the management of health care workers. Unlike managers in other industries, there is very little in the health care manager's sphere of influence that is static and constant. As discussed, the ability to deal effectively with change and conflict is paramount among these challenges. However, there are additional facets of health care management that require systematic, effective action, particularly at the line management level.

This chapter discusses the three most critical line management responsibilities: incremental performance planning, crisis management, and monitoring for potential unionization.

☐ Incremental Performance Planning

To ensure that employees achieve maximum performance, the manager must design a strategy of planning techniques that will optimize ongoing development of their knowledge and skills. One approach toward this goal is to use an incremental performance planning system. Such a system can be used with new and current employees, and with virtually anyone on the reporting staff. The system has three components:

- Selection of goals based on the job description, starting on day 1 of a new employee's service or, for current employees, on day 1 of a performance rating period
- Joint establishment of goals after six months of employment or, for current employees, after six months have passed in the performance rating period
- Joint establishment of new goals after one year of employment or at the end of the performance rating period

Initial Goal Setting

To build the basis for an incremental performance planning system, a sound job description program must first be in place. The job description should reflect at least 60 percent of what the employee does on a regular basis and at optimum 80 percent of the employee's critical responsibilities. With constant changes in health care work roles, 100 percent is not realistically attainable. A strong job description not only gives the manager clear goals with which to assess the employee, but more important, it gives the employee clear directions for the attainment of goals within a certain performance rating period. Conversely, job descriptions can be a de-motivator and source of dissatisfaction if they are obscure, fail to reflect the employee's responsibilities accurately, are outdated, or simply irrelevant to the employee's work role.

When the time comes to set initial goals—either on the first day of employment or the first day of the performance rating period—the manager will assign three to five concrete goals to the employee. The manager can draw these goals strictly from the major categories of a job description. The quantification of goals is essential to this process. All goals, whether from the job description or any other source, must be quantified using what is referred to as *performance quality indicators.* These include time, money, performance numbers, and percentages.

Time is any sequence or period in which the job should be accomplished or a specific project completed, and any other indicator that can be measured by time. For example, implementing a new process in accounts receivable might reduce the time over which a bill is collected. Or, implementing a computerized payroll system might reduce an employee's wait time for compensation. All important indicators that can be measured by time should be included in the incremental planning process.

The second performance quality indicator is *money.* This includes any expenditures involved in accomplishing a set of goals or the significant monetary figures attached to regular performance. For example, money considerations mandate that a staff member stays within a particular budget. Also, the monetary numbers might reflect a reduction of expenditures or a cost savings realized by the implementation of a new process. It is essential to tie money as well as time into the incremental planning process, because a goal achieved past a due date or regular responsibilities performed over budget are in fact examples of unacceptable performance.

The third performance quality indicator, *performance numbers,* is directed toward any significant progress or performance that can be measured by the reduction of a negative numerical category or the enhancement of a positive numerical category. For example, in the previous example of accounts receivable, performance might be measured as a reduction in days in accounts receivable or as an increase in the number of invoices processed per day. Or in the case of the payroll department, an enhancement in performance numbers might be indicated by an increase in the number of paychecks issued within a set time frame. Numerical indicators are very apparent to the manager, recognizable by the employee, and—once deemed fair by both parties—a sound touchstone for performance.

The fourth quality indicator is *percentages*. Virtually all aspects of the health care workplace involve some sort of percentage. The manager could use percentage indicators to encourage the employee to reduce a negative trend or increase a positive trend in performance. Percentages, like the other numerical indicators, can indicate group performance as well as individual performance. For example, if a manager uses performance quality indicators to set goals for a staff recruiter in the human resources department, the goals might include establishing a recruitment budget within the next three months, indicating the percentage of minority candidate interviews, reducing the number of days from the time a position opens to the time it is filled by a competent candidate, and implementing a job-posting system within a set length of time. By using the performance quality indicators, the employee has a clear idea of what performance is expected and has the opportunity to discuss various ways of accomplishing sound performance with the manager.

The goals are set up by the manager and expressed directly to the employee at the beginning of the performance rating period. These goals should be documented, preferably on a written performance evaluation plan, and expressed clearly to the employee. In addition to the goals, the performance evaluation plan should communicate the manager's intention to evaluate the employee's work personality, interpersonal skills, and team orientation, as well as any significant actions and critical contributions to the organization above and beyond the call of duty, as illustrated in the performance evaluation form in appendix B. The manager may also want to include with the plan some sort of employee development plan, as described in chapter 7 and illustrated in figure 7-2.

At this time the manager also indicates to the employee that after six months they will sit down and jointly review the progress made toward these goals. They will also formally review the nature and extent of the feedback and other communication that transpired between them during the first six months.

Six-Month Review

At the end of the first six months, the manager and employee once again discuss performance and review the goals set at the beginning of the performance rating period. If the employee has fulfilled those goals or is making reasonable and sound progress toward attaining them, the manager will take this opportunity to add more goals. On the other hand, if the employee is having difficulty with the original goals, the manager will offer specific guidance and assistance to ensure progress. At this point, the manager might also employ the crisis management action plan, which appears later in this chapter.

New goals at the six-month review should be drawn from the employee's attained expertise within the job role. As one demonstration of this new expertise, the employee should have the opportunity to submit a set of goals ahead of time to the manager for consideration. For example, one month before the six-month review, the employee might submit five to eight goals he or she would like added to the performance plan. Optimally, these would include activities the employee has seen as being essential to the job role, or goals and objectives the employee can address in the next six months. In the case of the staff recruiter, for example, these goals might include the implementation of a restructured interviewing system, the use of a candidate tracking form, the development of an employee referral program, or the restructuring of the basic recruitment process. All of these goals should be drawn not only from the employee's experience, but they should also utilize the employee's specific expertise and knowledge in his or her assigned area of the business.

By submitting these goals and objectives to the manager prior to the meeting, the employee gives the manager an opportunity to assess which goals are most important (for example, to choose the three goals that appear to be the most important and represent the largest potential contribution to the organization) and to rewrite the goals in a manner that utilizes performance quality indicators. When the time arrives for six-month review, the manager adds the three goals selected from the employee's original list to the performance plan. By doing so, the manager ensures that the employee is being challenged at a maximum level and being allowed to pursue a set of goals that are of interest to and intellectually engage him or her. Furthermore, these goals utilize a specific aspect of the employee's expertise and knowledge, and will now allow opportunity for further development of these skills.

In conducting the review session as a dialogue, the manager gives the employee a more participative role in the performance planning process and thus taps another source of motivation and inspiration for accomplishing job objectives. In "taking ownership" of these responsibilities, the employee feels a sense of pride and self-esteem in relation to these objectives, and will naturally take a strong interest in their accomplishment throughout the performance rating period. The net result is an employee who is well motivated and a health care organization that will benefit from the additional contributions of work and expertise.

One-Year Review

The final component of the incremental performance planning system is the one-year review at the end of the performance rating period. At this time, if the employee has attained all of the goals prescribed on day 1 and at the six-month interval, the employee again will have the opportunity to add some goals to the performance plan or to further develop specific areas of the job role. For example, the staff recruiter might "fine-tune" the goal of implementing a structured employee selection system to include department supervisors in addition to line managers. In addition, he or she might implement a community-based recruitment system to work in tandem with the employee referral program. Yet another example might be the use of a candidate tracking system that also indicates the performance of line managers relative to staff turnover and recruiting ability.

This final component allows a manager to set a clear course of performance for the upcoming year. It gives the individual employee a chance to participate actively in their job planning and in the organization's evaluation system, and to establish a line of communication with the manager that will preclude any ambivalence in addressing the manager in critical situations. Both the manager and the employee have a definite stake in what will occur and how the job will ultimately be accomplished.

Incremental performance planning is not only integral to progressive line management; it is also an important aspect of crisis management—in essence the most proactive form of crisis management. Incremental performance planning allows the manager and the employee to participate fully in the performance planning process, and thus to anticipate problems or changes that might dramatically affect the employee's performance and progress. Furthermore, it reinforces the lines of communication between the manager and the employee, and it sets a pattern for open discussion and clear communication. Both are valuable assets in dealing with crises on the job.

☐ Crisis Management

Despite all the planning that might occur in a health care workplace, and all the attention to detail paid by a manager relative to staff performance, certain crisis situations are bound to occur. The difference between an average health care manager and a superb one is the ability to deal positively with these situations and to engage the participation and quick action of staff not only to remedy the crisis but to ensure that the progress of the organization is not impeded. This is a difficult challenge, one that must be met realistically and on virtually a daily basis.

The Crisis Management System

The crisis management system consists of nine basic components:

1. Problem identification
2. Plan establishment
3. Preparation for action
4. Preparation for people interaction
5. Process commencement
6. Determination of possibilities, probabilities, and plausibilities
7. Prediction formulation
8. Plan review
9. Implementation of postcrisis measures

Problem Identification

Crises normally emerge from problems. Therefore, the first component of a crisis management system is to identify the specific problem (or problems) that caused the crisis. In essence, the manager and staff should get together and discuss the root of the problem. By making this a joint communicative effort, the manager gets the perspectives and specific input that only employees can provide and "sets the table" for the opportunity to get collective solutions and ideas toward addressing the problem.

In utilizing this component, the manager should strive to identify the root of the problem, its effect, and how the problem came to exist within the workplace. Identifying the problem, and understanding its cause and effects, eliminates ambiguity in addressing it successfully.

Plan Establishment

Establishing an initial plan is accomplished by asking a series of basic questions:

- How did the problem emerge?
- What can we do about it immediately?
- Which approach is the best way to go?
- How should we address the problem over the long term?
- Who should be involved in addressing the problem?
- Where should we start?

The only question *not* to ask is "Why does the problem exist?" This question should have been addressed when the problem was identified. Furthermore, at this point in time a solution is desired—not a second discussion on why the problem exists. In discussing a potential plan for addressing the problem, the manager asks for specific input and action plans from each employee for a full perspective on how the problem might be addressed successfully. Once this happens, staff members can detail their participation in addressing the problem and submit specific ideas and suggestions for their individual action.

Preparation for Action

By now, the problem has been identified and a basic overall plan has been established. However, the manager and staff must specifically determine who will play what role in addressing the problem. Furthermore, specific objectives will be assigned to each member of the staff and expectations/outcomes will be determined relative to each staff member's role in the solution process. All of the fiscal, operational, and human resources needed to resolve the problem are identified and enlisted in the effort to solve the crisis. Finally, time sequences are assigned to each particular phase of the plan, and general goals are established. At this point, a secondary plan (or a plan B) is established using the critical questions outlined previously.

Preparation for People Interaction

The entire range of human interaction is integral to the solution of the crisis. The manager controlling this problem-solving system should determine what segment of the employee population or customer population is affected most by the crisis, and how this crisis profoundly affects the basic "people aspect" of the health care organization's mission. Furthermore, the manager must ascertain which members of the reporting staff are the "people" most prepared, by virtue of their expertise and abilities, to deal advantageously with the crisis and bring it to a quick but effective solution. These people become the members of the crisis management team.

In addition, the manager must determine whether certain members of the reporting staff are not needed in the crisis management process but yet can play a secondary role. By giving full consideration to the "people quotient" in this equation, the manager is able to avert crisis.

Process Commencement

The manager and the crisis management team now move to the component of the crisis management system where the process of addressing the problem begins. Individual roles and time lines are confirmed and action begins in addressing the problem, and therefore the crisis.

The manager stays in close contact with all individuals addressing the problem and utilizes good communication, specifically feedback, as a main element in making this process successful. Once the process of addressing the crisis has been undertaken, it is essential for the manager to convene another meeting and to "regroup" staff in looking pragmatically at the process and how its initial stages are progressing. Next the manager makes a determination on whether to utilize the aforementioned plan B or maintain the course of the original plan. Also at this time, any minor adjustments can be made or additions to the plan can be incorporated in the entire process.

Determination of Possibilities, Probabilities, and Plausibilities

Once the process has begun, it is essential for the manager to discuss the possibilities, probabilities, and plausibilities that might occur as the individual department or crisis management team approaches the crisis itself. With the help of the subordinate staff, the manager must communicate the following:

- *Possibilities:* Anything that can occur as the team approaches the crisis, as well as all things that might occur on a regular basis because the crisis has become eminent.
- *Probabilities:* All things that are not only possible but that are likely to occur. This might include, for instance, individuals who become angered in the process of dealing with the crisis, a segment of the customer/patient population that might be affected by a change, or the probability of a goal being sacrificed or a secondary conflict occurring in dealing with a main crisis.
- *Plausibilities:* Plausibilities are potential occurrences that the crisis management team might believe to be eventualities at first glance, but in essence do not exist. The purpose of examining plausibilities is simply to make certain that nothing is "being taken for granted." This ensures that all "angles" are being examined and all action is being taken toward managing the crisis effectively.

Prediction Formulation

After reviewing the possibilities, probabilities, and plausibilities, the manager is able to predict the outcome of the crisis management effort. The manager is also able to predict the effect of the crisis resolution on the ongoing, "regular" flow of action in the workplace, such as whether the crisis would have a profound effect on how the department would be managed or administered from this point on, and whether the same crisis would recur.

Plan Review

Once the crisis is resolved, the manager reviews how it was managed, how effective the plan was, and what the future effect of the crisis and its management might be. This review considers, in retrospect, whether the crisis could have been avoided, or managed more effectively, or will occur again.

Implementation of Postcrisis Measures

To ensure that the crisis does not recur, the manager must take some specific steps following the completion of the crisis management process itself. First, the manager should share his or her perceptions of the situation with the staff as well as the supervisor, to make sure that all of the educational benefits of the crisis are realized. Second, the manager must implement fail-safe measures to prevent the crisis from occurring again. Third, the manager should underscore the organization's values and link the action taken toward the support of those values. Finally, the manager should use any existing or evolving means to assure employees that such crises can be handled almost routinely, and to provide the proper education, awareness, and training necessary toward that end.

Strong crisis management allows employees and managers alike in a progressive health care organization to be prepared to handle crisis situations effectively and efficiently. Furthermore, it minimizes risk to organizational effectiveness in that no department is taken "out of the action" due to a crisis situation.

Aspects of Interpersonal Crisis Management

In dealing with an interpersonal crisis between only two people, the manager must use a slightly different means for resolving a crisis quickly. He or she should consider six approaches to the crisis:

1. Ask questions.
2. Make a tough call.
3. Get input.
4. Balance outcome and mission.
5. React quickly and make timely decisions.
6. Respond appropriately to managerial requests.

These aspects can help ensure that the crisis is resolved and does not grow into destructive proportions that affect more of the work group.

Asking Questions

The manager must ask questions of employees relative to the problem that is occurring and what the effects of the crisis are. This is to determine the source of the crisis, how the crisis occurred, and, most important, what the employees think the resolution should be. In asking this third question, the manager will get data that can then be weighed and judged relative to a positive outcome.

Making the Tough Call

The manager must be able to make a tough call relative to resolving the situation despite its potential impact on the part of the employees. In a crisis situation, particularly one caused by interpersonal conflict, someone has to lose and someone has to win. The manager must seek fairness, not popularity. Ability to make a tough call reinforces the manager's credibility within the work group and the collective perception that he or she is fair and unbiased. This in turn will encourage most of the employees—at least the competent, highly motivated ones—to approach the manager with any interpersonal crisis situation.

Getting Input

In all crisis situations, notably those involving interpersonal conflict, the manager should seek as much input as possible. This includes not only asking questions but researching each situation and eliciting the opinions of individuals not directly involved in the crisis. This also includes other people who had similar jobs, or individuals who have contact with the employees involved in the crisis situation. The manager must be active in this role and maintain an objective stance.

Balancing Outcome and Mission

One guiding force throughout the resolution of an interpersonal crisis should be the manager's ability to balance what is fair and in sync with the institution's performance values against what is the quickest outcome. This means taking the time to have an extra discussion with the participants involved in the crisis, and to become as actively involved as possible.

Reacting Quickly and Making Timely Decisions

The manager must move as quickly and efficiently as possible in terms of collecting data, holding discussions with individuals in the work group, and any other action to resolve the situation. Moving slowly or too deliberately opens the floodgates for a variety of negative consequences and regressive outcomes.

Once all facts have been reviewed and the manager has gained as many data as possible from discussions and other fact-finding efforts, he or she must make timely decisions. Particularly in crisis situations it is important for the manager to make a quick decision, which hopefully can effect the most positive action for *both* individuals involved. Failure to take action quickly and firmly causes the affected employees not only to suffer a loss of optimum performance but also in the long term to find their own credibility and effectiveness within their work group hindered.

Responding Appropriately to Managerial Requests

A manager asked for information by another manager or pressed for a more detailed explanation of information relative to an interpersonal crisis must respond appropriately. This means using not only verbal communication, but in some cases, written communication. However, an undue amount of time must not be devoted to explaining or rehashing specific problems, such as within the context of a meeting not called for that purpose or at an unsuitable time. Particularly in the health care business setting, a manager must realize that sometimes the most compassionate response is "I'll get back to you shortly"—especially if his or her time is more urgently needed elsewhere.

All crisis management involves a set of skills that must be logically and pragmatically applied to the situation by the health care manager. No matter what level of the organization the manager administers, crisis management must be effective in defusing a potentially damaging set of circumstances, and efficient in the utilization of time, money, and effort to achieve the desired result. Only then can the manager's administrative resources truly be brought to bear in the maintenance of good relations among all employees.

☐ Responding to the Drive for Unionization in Health Care

Incremental performance planning, in concert with a solid approach to crisis management, can serve the organization well in ensuring a steady and positive flow of communication between employer and manager. When that communication breaks down, the climate may be ripe for workers to seek union representation. Despite cogent pro-union arguments, health care, because of its very nature, does not make clear the social benefits of health care unionization. Rather than approaching the issue from an antagonistic perspective, the remainder of this chapter looks at the entire issue with an emphasis on sound, progressive employee relations.

With the advent of the 1991 U.S. Supreme Court decision to allow the National Labor Relations Board (NLRB) the latitude to recruit and organize health care workers into union bargaining units, health care managers at all levels of the progressive organization must be aware of the potential impact of union organization, as well as some practical methods for addressing activities by unions.

Fundamentally, the Supreme Court decision has affected an already turbulent health care employee environment in several ways. For instance, the California Nurses Association and the Healthworkers Association of California, whose combined membership exceeds 55,000, are reported to be considering wholesale unionization, according to the August 24, 1991, issue of the *San Jose Mercury* newspaper. Nursing units across the country, as well as virtually all components of the health care organization personnel roster, could conceivably be organized into unions under the aegis of the five bargaining unit categories approved by the Supreme Court. In fact, skilled professionals in all areas could opt for unionization simply by filing the required petitions and mounting a membership campaign.

Union activity can create some challanges for the manager who is trying to maintain high levels of staff morale and productivity. The tension between employees who do and do not support the union, for example, could result in poor intradepartmental performance, a lack of communication, and other inhibitors of good performance. In another vein, the time spent on union campaigns could take time away from normal activities, as could postcampaign union activities.

If a drive is successful, introduction of the body of policies and procedures regarding union representation can prohibit open and direct communication between managers and their employees, as well as burdening the manager with time-consuming administrative tasks and procedures. Furthermore, a new employee may find that his or her indoctrination into the union can take precedence, in the minds of some employees, over the orientation and training of the new employee in the job position.

Asking Key Questions

There are several reasons why health care workers look on the union as a panacea for their problems on the job, some of which are real and valid, others of which are contrived and perceived. Some of the more reality-based reasons can be linked to inadequate compensation and benefit programs, lack of communication on the job, or mistreatment of employees. Basically, poor management at any level—if it can be substantiated and recognized by most members of a work unit—is the quickest and surest route to unionization in the health care setting. Close employee contact, open communication, and sound supervisory skills can go a long way in dissipating prounion sentiment, particularly circumstances in which a manager has inherited a disjointed, poorly motivated work group.

Open communication with employees regarding union representation can be fostered by asking such questions as:

- Are you willing to give a portion of your wages for union dues?
- Would you be pleased with a salary system that rewards time in the job and job level, but may not reward individual performance?
- Are you willing to accept more paperwork, rules, and regulations?
- Are you willing to spend more time in meetings, particularly during your free time away from the job?
- Do you have friends or family members who belong to unions? How happy are they with this form of representation?
- Are there ways we can work together to discuss directly your needs and concerns without the intervention of a third party?

Holding Monthly Staff Meetings

In addition to asking employees these key questions and supplying the facts about union representation, another strategy is to meet with staff once a month and delve into specific critical issues surrounding potential union sentiment. A strategy that is well formatted, forthright in nature, and timely in approach can go a long way toward addressing unionization activities as well as toward simply improving employee morale and maximizing staff input and communication. The most effective strategy for holding monthly meetings involves six basic steps:

1. Garner appropriate attendance.
2. Identify the major problems.
3. Ask what can be done now.
4. Ask what employees need from managers.
5. Ask employees for advice.
6. Determine the number-one improvement needed in the organization.

Garnering Appropriate Attendance

If the work unit is small, then every member should be included in these meetings, which can be called staff development meetings. If a larger work unit is involved, then one member from each segment of the work unit might be included, or several from each work team, so that a maximum number of representatives is between 12 and 15 participants. Each monthly meeting should consist of a different roster of people.

Identifying Major Problems

The opening query to the group should be "What major problems currently exist in the workplace?" Participants should be encouraged to openly discuss what problems are at hand, and the facilitator should encourage the participants to be as specific as possible so that generalities do not take precedence. Each problem should be addressed and potential solutions identified, particularly by the same individual who raised the problem. Then in turn each participant should have an opportunity to present a potential solution to the issue at hand.

The manager or discussion leader should make sure that positive solutions are discussed as much as possible, and that the emphasis is placed on categorizing issues by level of importance and pertinence to the daily workplace. To this end, it might be useful to have the participants rate each issue presented to them on a scale of 1–10, with 10 being most important and 1 being not that important at all.

Asking What Can Be Done Now

The group should then turn its attention to the question "What can be done in the next month?" This focuses attention on key issues that can be addressed succinctly and productively within a finite period of time. This question will elicit specific responses and ideas that can be acted on quickly, or at least responded to in a timely manner. This heightens employee trust in the process, as well as provides management with point-specific, pertinent feedback.

Asking about Employee Needs

Another question is "What do you need from us in management?" The key word in this query is *need*, as distinguished from *want*. On the one hand, all employees have certain needs if they are to conduct their respective job activities in a productive manner. On the other hand, all of us can cite a list of things we want from the workplace, many of which are simply not vital for the basic conduct of our jobs.

A list of needs from employees, particularly those needs commonly cited by more than one employee (or, for that matter, more than one group of employees) can be particularly illuminating for the management team conducting this process. Any action taken to meet these communicated needs can go a long way toward reinforcing managerial credibility and employee morale.

Asking Employees for Advice

Another useful question is "What would you do if you were in management?" This question might encourage some employees to suggest or imply the need for the manager's resignation, but hopefully the answers will provide a perspective not often seen in the subjective view of management. The answers could very well spark ideas that (1) management can immediately use but heretofore went unconsidered or (2) make management more aware of a small nuance of its conduct that has a major impact on employee motivation and the resultant productivity. Furthermore, the answers give the group facilitator an opportunity to explain any specific management issues that might be misunderstood by the employees or that might be "necessary evils" of the management process, such as a particular paperwork responsibility or a regulation outside management's control.

Determining the Number-One Need

Finally, the facilitator should elicit in each meeting what number-one improvement is needed in the collective viewpoint of the group. This could be a suggestion already mentioned by the group, or an additional suggestion arising from the combined opinion of the group. Additionally, an assortment of ideas might result from this question, giving the facilitator specific suggestions for action.

Importance of the Employee's Voice in the Workplace

The overall purpose of these suggestions for addressing union activity is to bring to the surface any underlying issues that might be adding to union sympathy, as well as to directly address apparent issues of concern among employees. By addressing these issues head on, and at least discussing the feasibility of various suggestions and solutions, the employees are provided with the participative voice that they might feel a union could provide. Furthermore, through the monthly meetings, a communication process is installed that can be employed regularly and effectively by management, provided feedback is given honestly to address employee concerns and provided appropriate follow-up is generated.

☐ Practical Applications

The following applications may serve as a starting point for improving the manager's ability to fulfill the three most critical line management functions:

1. Apply the incremental performance planning process to all new employees.
2. Incorporate the incremental performance planning process into the performance evaluation process of current employees.

3. Utilize the crisis management system with your own staff.
4. Educate your reporting team leaders and supervisors in utilization of the crisis management system.
5. Review past crisis situations. How would the crisis management system have assisted you in your efforts?
6. Utilize the key questions to address union sentiment.
7. Use monthly staff meetings to bolster employee relations.
8. Use any section of this chapter as part of an organizational training and development effort.
9. Share the information in this chapter with your peers and fellow managers in the interest of improving employee relations throughout the organization.
10. Add specific steps, as appropriate, to any strategy in the text.

Part Two

The Progressive Health Care Organization

Chapter 7

Progressive Human Resources Strategies

A key aspect of value-driven management is the examination of values with respect to the organization's human resources strategies. In that human resources by its very nature relates directly to the "human quotient" in a health care organization, it is only natural that special attention is directed toward this vital function. This chapter looks at the application of value-driven management to five essential areas of the human resources function.

In a sense, part of the responsibility of a solid human resources department in a health care organization is to safeguard the intents and objectives of value-driven management strategies as they relate to employees and managerial personnel. The very charter of a human resources department is to increase the effectiveness and efficiency of the organization's personnel. Because each one of the major functions of a human resources department—organizational development, training and development, compensation and benefits, recruitment, and employee relations—is important to an employee's daily work life, it is essential that this department take the lead in ensuring that high ethical management standards are an integral part of the personnel administration process. It is equally important for the organization to focus closely on its human resources functions, particularly in how that department reflects the values held by the organization's management.

☐ Organizational Development

Organizational development is the human resources function that provides the impetus for organizational growth, cohesiveness, and interactive strength. Organizational development is the focus of human resources that seeks to gain a synergistic effect from the contributions of several organizational components, and from the entire complement of individuals working within the organization. In health care, this is particularly essential. A health care organization must act as a cohesive unit and provide its employees with legitimate, visible means of upward progressive and professional growth within the organization. It is the responsibility of the human resources department to identify opportunities to enhance organizational growth, and to maintain a system that will encourage progressive development of the organization's human resources.

Many leading national health care organizations have large organizational development departments that specifically focus on internal promotions and personal development among its various hospitals and health care institutions. However, the importance of such a strategy is underscored when smaller chains and individual institutions are also observed employing organizational development as part of their ongoing strategy for growth.

For example, the Bon-Secours Health System employs an organizational development strategy from its national office in Columbia, Maryland. However, at its leading hospitals, such as the Bon-Secours Hospital in Grosse Point, Michigan, an organizational development department is also in place. The intelligence of this action is evidenced by the low rate of turnover, high frequency of internal promotions, and organizationwide readiness of this facility. Not coincidentally this organization employs a strong system of ethical human resources practices, including a performance evaluation that scores the individual employee performance in ethics-related work responsibilities. (See chapter 3 and appendix B for an introduction to value-driven performance evaluations.)

Communication System

The first aspect of organizational development is improvement of the facility's communication system. The health care organization has a responsibility to its employees to communicate many facets of its operations in a clear and concise manner. Major policies should be clearly delineated and expressed to the employees, from initial orientation through all phases of the employee's work life. This particularly relates to any change that might occur in the environment; for example, in organizational policy, operational procedure, or introduction of new programs into the system. Many progressive health care organizations accomplish this goal through a newsletter, especially in smaller community hospitals, which often publish a monthly newsletter for both employees as well as customer/patients. A newsletter keeps relevant personnel and the customer community aware of new programs, facility improvements, advancements in programs and services provided, or any other information of interest to readers.

A strong communication system in a health care institution is important for several reasons. First, the organization has an ethical commitment to relay essential information to its employees. Because the employee is an important foundation component, it is also "good business" to keep the employee as informed as much as possible, and as appropriately as possible, of any significant events or actions taken by the organization.

Second, gossip or hearsay is perhaps one of the most detrimental outcomes of human interaction. A strong organizational communication system precludes the festering of gossip in the workplace and keeps a factual frame of reference in a prominent position in the employees' and customer/patients' perceptions.

Third, a strong organizational communication system also demonstrates a high degree of compassion for both the customer community as well as the individual employee. It implicitly expresses a degree of respect for the employee, a sense of importance toward the employee, and the opportunity for the employee to actively participate in any significant organizational action.

Management System

Another aspect of organizational development is the management system, that is, the type of power an organization exerts, from the executive suite down to the "low end of the totem pole." The style of management employed by an organization is in and of itself an expression of the organization's values and its adherence to, and respect for, an ethically based approach to management.

To demonstrate how values are reflected in the organization's approach to management, it is useful to examine three types of management systems that could be developed and utilized in health care organizations—the autocracy, the pyramid organization, and management by committee.

The Autocracy

In an autocratic management system, one individual, usually a strong CEO or administrator, makes the majority of decisions for the organization. The system generally discourages input from other members of the organization, which has the effect of prohibiting significant employee interaction and leaves the responsibility for critical judgments and the setting of organizational direction to one individual. In an autocracy it is common for individuals to believe they are victims of a dictatorship and have little lasting motivation besides money or financial reward. This style of leadership can be found in some smaller community hospitals, entrepreneurial health care organizations, or smaller specialty institutions.

An autocracy may create the impression that the organization has little regard for the individual worker or manager. Turnover can be very high and innovation is almost nonexistent. The reason for this is quite simple. The individuals who stay at the organization for a long time are encouraged to do only what is required by their job description. Furthermore, they have no incentive to be creative or inventive. This will eventually cripple the progress of the organization because no new thoughts or progressive suggestions will be provided out of fear of termination on the part of the individual employees or managers.

The Pyramid Organization

The pyramid organization has a CEO with a staff of associate administrators or vice-presidents representing the major functional areas of the organization. In this setting, individuals can make suggestions or provide input through their respective chain of command until it reaches the top decision-making stratum. The pyramid system is essentially a good structure for most hospital settings. It allows for significant interaction among members and encourages the infusion of creative suggestions and progressive thought through the proper channels to the executive decision-making level.

A pyramid organization embraces good ethical standards. The organization demonstrates to its employees a desire to hear their ideas and perceptions, and to consider their suggestions for taking action. Sometimes, however, the organization might stifle creative thought somewhere along the organizational lines of report; though in general, the pyramid system of management gets employees involved and, from the other direction, establishes clear-cut lines of report for organizational direction and employee motivation and performance.

Management by Committee

Management by committee is seen in organizations that feel *too* much of a commitment toward employee involvement in managing the institutions. In this type of organization, any particular health care management issue or organizational dynamic is reviewed by a committee. Rather than maintaining a sense of a representative democracy, the organization forms a committee of staff members and employees to review each and every issue. This type of management is prominent in government organizations and in organizations with a large union membership.

The ethical ramification of management by committee is that a commitment to the employee's welfare is being fulfilled, but that of the customer/patient is being neglected. Because such a system usually stalls action and prohibits quick reaction to a situation or set of circumstances (which is mandatory in a health care organization), the needs of the customer/patient are secondary to those of the employee.

The organization must foster a management system that takes into equal consideration the needs of the customer/patient as well as the motivational and professional needs of the employee. As demonstrated in an earlier section of this chapter, the success of that system depends in large measure on strong communication channels throughout the organization.

Organizational Culture

Another aspect of organizational development is the culture a health care organization reflects through its actions and statements. An organization's culture and personality should reflect several factors.

First, the organization should have a strong regard for the individual rights of all employees. It should realize that the employee is the most important factor in any successful organization, paramount to any equipment, financial resources, or state-of-the-art buildings. The organization must be adaptable in dealing with a variety of employees and respect the individual dignity of each and every employee.

Second, the organization should convey, particularly in its mission statement, a set of organizational values similar to those described in chapter 3. How the organization expresses its culture and standards of conduct is as important as the standards themselves. The Unitek Corporation of Los Angeles, for example, has a novel approach to publishing its mission statement; it has it printed and encased in an employee keychain that is coated with the same material used in many of the facility's orthodontic products. This way, all employees are reminded of the mission statement when they start their cars up in the morning to drive to work, and then again at the end of the day. Other organizations incorporate their organizational charter and cultural objectives into their performance evaluation systems and training programs, as will be shown later in this chapter.

Organizational Charter

As further reinforcement to its organizational culture, the institution should have a strong organizational charter, which is a summary of the basic objectives and mission. For example, one prominent Catholic health care organization states as its mission "To provide stellar health care to those in need in the best traditions of Christianity." As far as being problematic for non-Christian customer/patients, the commitment to "Christian care" has the same connotation of standards of high quality as a Jewish deli or a Persian rug.

Organizational Personality

Organizational culture needs to be a reflection of the organization's personality, which is a composite of four factors: a strong employee attitude or orientation that puts the patient/customer at the top of the organization's chart, a good set of people skills among all employees, a strong managerial aptitude, and a team orientation. These factors of personality should apply to all aspects of the organization's human resources function, notably in the areas of employee selection and performance evaluation.

Organizational Action

The actions the organization undertakes must reflect both its charter and personality. For example, from an ethical standpoint, are all employees given the opportunity to succeed, without regard for cultural background or socioeconomic differences? Has the organization always sought to provide optimum health care and been zealous in making the best use of its allocated resources? Does most of the "press" generated by both the media and the organization reflect sound ethics? Finally, does the individual employee believe he or she is part of a strong organization committed to helping others in a sound, ethical manner?

Industrial psychologists from Maslow to Drucker have stressed the importance of the individual's perception of the organization. An individual in any industry is highly motivated by the belief that he or she is part of a winning, successful entity. Therefore, a value-driven approach to organizational development not only will help the overall ethical "health" of an organization, but also help to motivate each individual to contribute positively to the organization.

☐ Training and Development

The human resources subfunction of training and development is essential to the ethical management of a health care organization. The objectives of training and development are to increase organizational readiness, progressively develop the professional abilities and technical acumen of employees, and provide growth opportunities for all members. As such, training and development programs have an innate responsibility to strengthen human resources for future growth and progressive business development.

To reduce the turnover attributable to a perceived lack of promotional opportunities and developmental programs, a progressive facility has the ethical responsibility to have in place a system that gives employees a chance to participate in activities that will enhance their long-term professional development, that is, to be the best they can be. Furthermore, from a business perspective, the organization should develop existing personnel in order to avoid the high cost of outside recruitment and other costly effects of turnover. By formulating a training strategy that helps maximize employee performance, a personnel planning and development program that charts the promotion opportunities for deserving employees, and an internal promotion program that prepares employees for opportunities within the organization over the long term, the organization lives up to its ethical commitment to its employees and gains a distinct business benefit of greater organizational readiness and development.

Personnel Planning

As indicated in the preceding section, an organization's personnel planning system builds on its system of performance evaluation and charts promotion opportunities for the individual employee. An organizational chart for assessing promotability (as illustrated in figure 7-1) and a training

Figure 7-1. Organizational Chart for Assessing Promotability

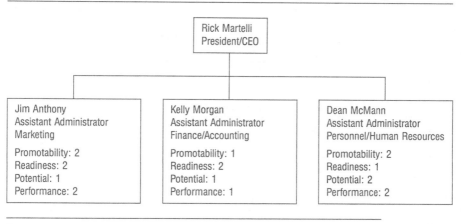

Rick Martelli
President/CEO

Jim Anthony
Assistant Administrator
Marketing

Promotability: 2
Readiness: 2
Potential: 1
Performance: 2

Kelly Morgan
Assistant Administrator
Finance/Accounting

Promotability: 1
Readiness: 2
Potential: 1
Performance: 1

Dean McMann
Assistant Administrator
Personnel/Human Resources

Promotability: 2
Readiness: 1
Potential: 2
Performance: 2

Key:

1. Long-term promotability
   Immediate readiness
   High potential
   Stellar performance

2. Well-placed promotability
   1–3-year readiness
   Good potential
   Good performance

3. Limited promotability
   2–5-year readiness
   Limited potential
   Conditional performance

and development plan (figure 7-2) can help an organization prepare for future growth and implement a backup system for all significant positions.

The personnel planning system demonstrates the organization's commitment to the employee's future, its interest in the employee's development, and the value the organization places on individual employee contribution.

A strong training system utilizes internal and external educational opportunities in assisting employees to grow as professionals. External opportunities include seminars presented by various professional groups, accreditation bodies, and management and professional associations. Such opportunities can also be found at local educational institutes, health care management conferences, and community-generated educational forums that provide insight and knowledge for the modern health care professional.

Figure 7-2. Personnel Training and Development Plan

Employee Name: _____

Employee Position: _____

In-Service Training Planned:

	Activity	Rationale/Benefit	Timing
a.	_____	_____	_____
b.	_____	_____	_____
c.	_____	_____	_____

External Training Planned:

	Course	Rationale/Benefit	Timing
a.	_____	_____	_____
b.	_____	_____	_____

On-the-Job Training and Development Planned:

	Assignment	Rationale/Benefit	Timing
a.	_____	_____	_____
b.	_____	_____	_____
c.	_____	_____	_____

The benefit of outside training is the exposure the employee receives to the methods employed by other organizations and fellow managers in other professional environments. In attending such programs, the employee is receiving a pat on the back from the organization and is being shown that the organization is willing to invest tangibly in his or her future.

Internal training programs, popularly known as in-service programs, are equally effective if employed correctly. Perhaps the most progressive system of internal training and development in the United States is the Progressive Management Development Program (PMDP) of the Jane Phillips Medical Center (JPMC) near Tulsa, Oklahoma.

Spearheaded by hospital CEO Larry Minden and directors Tomme Moore and Henry Hobbs, the program provides JPMC's managers with perspectives on meaningful topics ranging from employee selection and performance evaluation to conflict management and productivity. These subjects are taught by national experts in each subject area and presented to a core group of over 75 of the institution's managers and supervisors. Although the program is somewhat costly, the financial benefit of an increased organizational readiness in these areas, the expression of commitment to the employees attending the programs, and the overall benefit of enlightenment far outweigh program costs. Furthermore, the cost of sending more than 75 people to an outside seminar with this venue indeed would be staggering.

If an internal seminar encourages employees to hire candidates who do not cost the organization large sums in turnover costs, civil action suits, or any other expenses inherent in poor selection, the program's financial benefits are easily realized. Furthermore, the ethical commitment to employee development is demonstrated clearly. In the case of the PMDP program, the organization's culture, charter, and basic objectives are driven home by the themes presented in each program. By including managers and supervisors as well as executives, the entire JPMC community is given the opportunity to participate, reap the benefits of progressive education, and develop professionally in accordance with the demands and challenges of the health care environment of one of the nation's largest cities.

The range of training topics a manager or supervisor is exposed to via external or internal training programs reflects the ethical commitment to employees. Programs dealing in the basic management process—from supervisory skills to personnel selection, and from performance evaluation to conflict management—underscore the importance of ethical management practices relative to the human resources of the organization. For example, programs dealing in stress management, a most popular topic for the 1990s in health care management, reflect a commitment to the individual employee's personal health. Programs dealing in equal

opportunity and facets of affirmative action can exemplify the organization's ethical commitment to fair play among employees and the manner in which they conduct business.

Technical training programs show an ethical commitment to the
development of technical acumen and professional knowledge among
employees. Furthermore, the health care worker given instruction on
the latest techniques in his or her discipline is likely to feel a sense of
allegiance to the organization for providing these opportunities. Whether
conducted on-site or off-site, these programs can be delivered in group
settings, as well as through computer-assisted instruction, self-managed
programs (such as programmed instruction), or specific educational cur-
riculums provided by local educational institutions and technical schools.

Besides training seminars and other obvious educational opportunities, the organization's ethical commitment to training and development can be demonstrated in other ways. First, the use of internships,
that is, on-the-job training through a local educational institution or a
professional association, is a terrific way of fostering a sense of allegiance in a prospective employee or one who is new to health care. Internships also can be an effective motivator for a professional already working
for the organization. On-the-job training might include cross-training,
where an individual works in another department, equipment training,
or training in an operational procedure.

Second, a reading program that incorporates a list of books or publications that enhance professional development is an often-overlooked
but highly efficient training and development device. With a planned
reading program the manager can increase the employee's awareness
of a particular area as well as assist the employee personally in gaining
competency in a given technical area.

Finally, delegation, if done skillfully so as to enhance the employee's
knowledge and exposure to a wider set of responsibilities, can be an excellent development strategy. It also gives the manager the opportunity to
personally supervise the employee's training and development program
while grooming a backup for the manager's position.

Whether it be on-the-job training, a reading program, or the delegation of responsibility, training and development are effective motivators and concrete evidence of a facility's ethical commitment to the
employee and to the mission of health care.

Enhancement Steps

An organization can take several steps quickly and efficiently in the health
care environment to enhance training and development efforts ethically.
First, an employee survey should be taken to examine current programs
and to elicit ideas of what types of training and development are needed.

Second, the human resources staff should seek the best possible training and development programs for presentation to the organization's employees. These could include "off-the-shelf" generic programs that are readily available from various training and development organizations. They could also include customized programs, tailored specifically by training and development staff (in a large institution) or by the human resources staff.

Third, the health care organization should seek training opportunities that are as specific to the health care environment as possible. Although some lessons can be learned from other industries, the health care environment is unique in terms of its pace, various pressures, and products and services. Therefore, a progressive organization will strive to employ training and development techniques and course presenters who have specific knowledge of the health care business arena. After all, the ethical commitment to health care employees is to provide instruction that will assist them in their *specific* fields of expertise. Use of materials or instructors having little relevance to or knowledge of specific nuances of the health care environment can be insulting and seem merely as a cosmetic appeal to employees.

As emphasized earlier, progressive health care training and development demonstrates ethical commitment to employee growth and development, fosters allegiance among organizational members, is a sign of respect for the dignity of all employees, and helps reinforce the organization's charter and desired cultural norms. In a larger business sense, sound training and development strategies prepare human resources for future growth and progressive action on behalf of the organization.

For a review of the organizational development strategies presented in this chapter, and for further strategies that may prove useful to your organization's human resources function, refer to the summaries and planning work sheets in appendix D.

□ Compensation and Benefits

Perhaps the most visible segment of a health care organization's human resources activities is compensation and benefits. Along with the desire to help fellow human beings, to practice a humanistic trade, and to be part of a winning organization, health care workers still regard money as a paramount motivator. Therefore, fair play and fair pay should underlie all aspects of a health care organization's compensation and benefits policy.

Job Analysis, Description, and Evaluation

A health care organization's compensation system is based on three essential factors. First, every job must undergo *analysis* so that the compensation system takes into account how the job is perceived by the organization in terms of its specific elements, its daily responsibilities, and its importance to the overall organization.

Second, most health care organizations are somewhat remiss in the maintenance of accurate and realistic *job descriptions.* In order for a job to be properly gauged with a compensation level, a job description must be clear, thorough, and accurate in reflecting the daily responsibilities of the job. Lack of an accurate job description is an organizational breach of ethical commitment to the employee to properly recognize and reward his or her contribution to the organization's success.

The third factor of a compensation system, *job evaluation,* calls for the organization to review the job analysis and the job description to ascertain a fair level of compensation. The job evaluation can be performed using a number of tools:

- *Ranking system:* The employee's rank within the organization is established on a lineal basis relative to the nature of the organization's services and the employee's importance to the organization.
- *Classification:* The job is placed at a certain level or designated a certain grouping based on the nature of the primary work activity and number of tasks undertaken in a typical day.
- *Factor analysis:* The organization assesses the difficulty of a job or the skills needed to perform it successfully.
- *Point system:* An organization assigns a number of points to a job based on an amalgamation of factors from the three preceding job evaluation tools.
- *Policy:* This refers to the importance of the individual in the organizational hierarchy in terms of setting organizational policy, such as key strategic planning or significant organization programs and direction.
- *Comparable worth:* Wage surveys and other market data are used to ascertain a salary level based on the individual's professional worth as deemed by societal norms, business trends, and other external factors.

A strong ethical compensation system will seek to employ a job evaluation scheme incorporating as many of these tools as possible. For example, the nature of a floor nurse's contribution to the organization (ranking), the skills required, the nurse's marketability in the job sector, and the nurse's handling of critical incidents and high-demand situations are all essentials that must be considered in evaluating the job fairly. Simply put, the organization has an ethical commitment to reward the floor nurse for the entirety of his or her contribution to the organization. There is no surer de-motivator than an employee's not being compensated at a level he or she feels is just. Therefore, thoughtful job evaluations based on thorough job analyses and accurate job descriptions are vital to maintain a high level of motivation among employees, as well as to maintain equity within the organization's compensation system.

Compression

Lack of equity is referred to by human resources specialists as compression. *Compression* occurs when some individuals are paid a higher compensation than others who have essentially the same responsibilities to the organization—or even hold the same job position. Compression issues often arise in large national organizations where, for example, a worker in Cincinnati is paid less than a worker in New York City, due to regional differences in the cost of living. In this case, the compression is fair because the individual in New York City works and lives in an environment that has a higher cost of living. However, if two health care professionals have the same position in St. Louis but are paid at two different levels, this is a problem of compression. A health care organization, then, must consider several factors regarding compression and its ethical ramifications.

To begin with, seniority must be rewarded, as must the degree of expertise an individual brings to a job. Two individuals with the same job but with different levels of expertise and seniority status within the organization logically should be paid different compensations. Obviously, the employee with the higher seniority and greater expertise should be the better performer. However, if the worker with less expertise and lower seniority status performs at a higher level, then he or she should be compensated accordingly. When compression becomes a negative issue, it is usually due to disproportionate compensation based on issues other than performance, seniority, or expertise—for instance, favoritism, sexism, racism, or other unethical criteria.

Incentive-Based Compensation

The incorporation of an incentive-based compensation system into the human resources function is extremely vital to a health care organization. In fact, this has become one of the hottest issues in health care human resources strategic management. An incentive-based compensation system rewards stellar performance, that is, the attainment of a set group of goals and objectives and work contributions to the organization above and beyond the call of duty.

Incentive-based compensation systems are found most commonly at the executive level, because usually these individuals have already in place a MBO (management by objective) system. However, the organization can demonstrate its firm ethical commitment to employees at all levels of the organization if every individual is allowed to participate in a bonus scheme or incentive-based compensation system appropriate for their particular work activities. Such a system also serves as an innovative motivational tool.

Wage Surveys

The use of wage surveys is essential to the ethical composition of a health care organization's compensation programs. Wage surveys should be conducted by the hospital's human resources department, which should contact human resources directors at 6–12 other area providers to compare wage information in various occupational fields (nursing, dietary, physical therapy) and other essential components of a health care organization. This information should then be used to adjudicate the wage structure and salary administration of the hospital. This information, if favorable to the organization, should be publicized to all members of the organization as evidence of the facility's commitment to equitable compensation. If the information is not favorable to the organization, steps should be taken to increase the compensation levels, if at all appropriate and feasible, in order to decrease the likelihood of turnover.

Nonmonetary Rewards

A final aspect of compensation and benefits relates directly to rewards other than salary dollars. A sound benefits program should incorporate a pension system, retirement plans, medical and life insurance benefits, and a savings program.

Some organizations, notably those in the Northeast, have used a system of "matching dollars" for their savings programs. This is a very intelligent as well as ethically sound concept, which rewards the employee over time and shows loyalty on behalf of the employer. For every dollar an employee saves, 20 cents is contributed by the organization. At the end of five years, using a 20-cent-per-year increment, the employee is being "matched" dollar for dollar by the organization. This encourages the maximum employee performance, a long-term commitment by the employee, and a reward by the employer for employee allegiance. After reaching the maximum dollar-for-dollar level after five years, other rewards, such as an employee purchase program, an increase in vacation days, or other incentives, are provided.

For years this form of compensation has been used by a number of large corporations outside health care as part of their vesting programs. Applied by progressive health care organizations such as Bon-Secours, it is not only a great motivator but a reflection of a strong ethical commitment to long-term performance. The stronger a health care benefits package is—from insurance to savings to pension/retirement programs—the stronger the long-term commitment on the part of the employee to the employer is likely to be. The outcome is higher monetary rewards for the employee, and long-term fiscal stability and optimum performance for the employer.

☐ Recruitment

The recruitment and selection strategies utilized by a health care organization's human resources department have ethical ramifications to both the internal and external environments of an organization. From the outside, the manner in which an organization recruits and selects employees reflects its commitment to quality and a high standard of health care provision. From the viewpoint of current employees, the type of new employee recruited by the organization shows its commitment to building a stronger team and to maintaining excellence in the health care business setting.

The human resources department, as well as all line managers and executives involved in the recruitment process, have an ethical responsibility to attract the most qualified people possible. Managers and executives have the same responsibility to existing employees to bring qualified, highly motivated people into the fold.

From a public relations standpoint—the most important angle—the recruiter and hiring manager have a responsibility to the outside applicant to make a fair decision based on objective criteria and ability to perform job tasks. Nothing is worse for the reputation of a health care organization than the perception that its hiring practices are unfair or biased.

Before it even considers recruiting from the outside a progressive health care organization will investigate all internal applicants for the job. This is predicated on the facility's having (1) a good job-posting system for announcing openings and (2) a policy of encouraging current employees to apply. These prerequisites not only give ethical veracity to the organization's commitment to internal development, but they also save outside recruiting dollars and prevent high turnover resulting from employee perception of a lack of opportunities.

In recruiting from the outside, the human resources department should seek to establish a variety of sources for any given opening. By using the media, professional journals, and schools and technical institutions, the recruiter can get a wide variety of candidates with an assortment of technical backgrounds and socioeconomic roots. This helps in fostering a plurality of employee population and ensuring the best possible candidate for the position. A good recruitment strategy, which has tremendous relevance for value-driven management, is employee referral.

Employee Referral

Employee referral is a system by which, following the unsuccessful attempt at an internal search, a job position is posted and a "bounty" is placed on the position. This "bounty" might consist of an established amount of money, an additional day or two off, or a product from the employee purchase program. To receive this reward, an employee must recommend to the human resources department an individual who ultimately is hired.

An employee referral system taps into the employee's knowledge of potential candidates, encourages the employee to take ownership for filling vital job openings, and cuts down drastically on recruitment costs. It also demonstrates organizational values such as forthrightness, allegiance, and other norms of behavior desired by a progressive health care organization.

A proviso for handling employee referrals in an ethical manner is that each candidate must be treated fairly, given a full opportunity to interview, and have his or her application handled efficiently, whether hired or not. This treatment includes relaying the final decision to the applicant and providing a brief candid reason as to why he or she was or was not hired. A thank you letter should be sent to both the candidate and the referring employee for their efforts. The employee's letter should encourage him or her to participate in future referral activities.

Interviewing

The interviewing process should be as objective as possible, and a structured approach to interviewing will help the organization ensure that its criteria for selection are fair, that the questions asked in the interview are equitable, and that its decision is made on the candidate's ability to do the job. A subjective interviewing process—using ineffective questions, biased decision-making rationale, or inconclusive evidence—can only harm the organization. Furthermore, it violates the ethical responsibility to qualified candidates and to the facility's objective of superb health care provision.

Because the selection standards should reflect the organization's charter, the interviewer should seek evidence that the candidate's work personality is congruent with the organization's values, mission, and culture. Evidence should be based on objective fact and past performance, not on subjective opinion or obliging behavior on the part of the candidate. The interview questions in appendix A may serve to help the interviewer identify the most appropriate candidates for a given position.

A variety of managers should be included on the interviewing slate and participate in the hiring process—the human resources specialist, the reporting manager for the open position, and, ideally, the executive to whom that manager is accountable. The human resources specialist should verify references and conduct an in-depth interview relative to the work personality and overall potential of the candidate. The hiring manager should focus on the individual's technical merits and professional qualifications for the job. The supervising manager (executive) should evaluate the candidate's potential to fit into the organizational culture. By getting a variety of viewpoints, the ethical commitment to the organization to make an optimum decision is fulfilled, and the responsibility to the candidate to fully present the qualifications for the position is satisfied.

Outplacement

Outplacement, that is, assisting terminated employees with finding new employment, has become an unfortunate reality in the health care field. However, even this final activity can serve to underscore an organization's commitment to its employees. Outplacement includes counseling, help with preparing resumes, instruction on how to interview, and an initial list of prospective new employers. Outplacement can be conducted by firms that specialize in the health care setting or by the terminating facility's own human resources department. In addition to offering assistance to those affected by the termination, outplacement may reassure remaining workers who observe the process. It also fulfills an ethical commitment to the customer community. Finally, outplacement is smart business in that the organization's image as a humane employer is enhanced.

☐ Employee Relations

Employee relations is the day-to-day treatment of employees, notably among the hourly ranks, by the organization and its management. The health care organization has an ethical commitment to treat each employee fairly, that is, to provide a safe workplace in which opportunities exist equally for everyone.

As touched on in an earlier chapter, many organizations, as part of their employee relations activities, charge the human resources department with implementing surveys—climate surveys, wage surveys, turnover studies, organizational needs analysis, and others—to gain pertinent

information on employee morale and needs. In terms of the organization's commitment to value-driven management, the intent of a survey
must be clear, so as not to arouse suspicion about "hidden agendas."
Such clarity helps to garner an effective and candid response.

The manner in which the surveys are scored must be clearly stated,
and upon conclusion of the study the results should be published. Both
actions communicate to employees that their opinions were registered
and eliminate fear of being singled out for expressing their opinions.

Finally, any significant action that takes place as a result of the survey should be clearly described before it is implemented, and any
promises made should be fulfilled. If there is no response to the actions
indicated by the survey, or if the survey provokes excessive emotional
response, not only is the trust between the organization and the
employee compromised, but no positive business effect is realized.

Employee Health Programs

The environment in which an employee works is key to employee relations. For example, because stress is such a major factor in the health
care workplace, an organization should take steps to mitigate the effects
of stress as much as possible. One step would be to provide employee
health programs, such as fitness programs, paid for by the employer.
The organization demonstrates concern for the employee's health while
at the same time minimizing sick days and resulting downtime.

The organization should also encourage employees to suggest ways
to improve safety and health within the workplace. Moreover, the
employer should respond to these suggestions, whenever possible, with
corrective action. For example, a smaller midwestern hospital did not
have the resources to provide an on-site workout center for its employees
but was willing to help establish an employee health program. Several
employees suggested through the suggestion box that the hospital enter
into an agreement with a local fitness club. In pursuing this course of
action, not only did the administration provide employees with an opportunity to maintain good health and fitness, it also gave a large amount
of business to the local customer community and demonstrated an ethical
commitment to both the community as well as members of the
organization.

Grievance Handling

Part of employee relations is handling grievances. In a unionized situation, responsibility for handling grievances falls mainly to the union
representative and management. In a nonunion environment, this
responsibility falls to the human resources manager, the employee, and

the manager. In either case, evidence must be collected in an honest manner, and the values of decency, dignity, and forthrightness must be invoked in constructing a resolution. No favoritism should be shown, and corrective action should be taken as quickly as possible. As a motivator, the integrity of a just system for discipline and grievance resolution is essential.

A comprehensive disciplinary system consists of warning(s), probation, and, if necessary, termination. An employee should receive a verbal warning when he or she does something that is detrimental to the conduct of the organization or the department. The verbal warning should be followed by a written warning, copies of which should go to both the human resources department and the supervising executive.

The second disciplinary step is probation. If the employee fails to correct the offending conduct or repeats an unacceptable behavior, he or she should be put on probation per a letter that allows three months in which to remedy the problem.

The third step, failing probation and warnings, is termination. The employee terminated for cause should be terminated quickly and given a severance package of only two weeks' pay. This sends a clear statement to other employees that inappropriate behavior will not be tolerated and that the consequences will be dealt with fairly and expediently. This helps to uphold the ethical responsibility of the manager to the organization to compensate and reward only good performance as well as the ethical responsibility of the organization to the customer community to maintain a strong, positively motivated, value-driven work force.

Performance Evaluations

A key to rewarding employees, fostering good employee relations, and taking appropriate disciplinary action is the performance evaluation. As demonstrated in chapter 6, a strong criterion-based performance evaluation is the order of the day for a progressive health care organization.

To review, a performance evaluation program should embrace the following mandates:

- Rely on specific job criteria
- Incorporate work personality characteristics
- Utilize clear, understandable forms
- Establish future goals
- Articulate a training plan
- Provide continuous feedback throughout the grading period with the employee
- Allow for appropriate employee participation and feedback
- Be relevant to compensation administration and incentives

In reviewing these fundamentals, the health care organization can ensure fulfillment of its ethical responsibility to employees in terms of just rewards and progressive human resources development.

Sensitive Situations

Finally, any sensitive situations in which the human resources department engages relative to the actions of individual employees must be handled ethically and within prescribed legal boundaries. For example, an employee assistance program as it relates to a particular employee should be handled in a manner that strikes a judicious balance between necessary disclosure and the employee's right to privacy and confidentiality. This means clarifying the delicate line between respect for an employee's dignity and a supervisor's "need to know." This is particularly true in the United States and Canada, where individual employee rights are paramount, especially in the health care setting. Adherence to the values described in chapter 3 will help the institution guarantee preservation of these rights.

☐ Practical Applications

The human resources function is the area of value-driven health care management in which the "rubber hits the road." The manner in which a company treats employees, rewards performance, and provides for long-term development makes a loud statement regarding its personality, culture, and objectives. As demonstrated by the premier health care organizations cited herein, a successful facility incorporates stellar people management skills. As is often the case, ethical management means good business.

Use the following practical applications as a starting point for improving the degree to which the human resources function in your institution reflects the principles of value-driven management:

1. Review the specific strategies for personnel development and staff investment in appendix D.
2. Implement a value-driven approach to the management of human resources within your area of responsibility.
3. Reinforce your mission objectives by utilizing the specific interviewing questions (cues) in appendix A as part of your interviewing strategy.
4. Involve your reporting managers and staff in the identification and use of programs delineated in the chapter as part of your ongoing management development process.

5. Set up a training and development plan for all staff members, as illustrated in the chapter.
6. If you are a senior executive, conduct an audit of your human resources function and implement new strategies with your human resources staff. Review all organizationwide applications with board members and, when appropriate, elicit their involvement.
7. Use this chapter as a discussion point in both management retreats and planning sessions.
8. Garner employee opinion and input relative to the strategies outlined in this chapter.

Chapter 8

Case Study: Progressive Human Resources Management

This chapter reviews a "real-life" situation involving the progressive development of a key staff member, from the point of selection to the completion of the first year on the job. The objective is to understand how the value-driven criteria in chapter 3 are applied to the staff selection process, as well as how a personnel development plan and several other human resources strategies are instituted within the new executive's first year of employment.

□ Case Situation

During the past seven years, the CEO/administrator of Delaware City Hospital (DCH) has been able to build a competent and well-versed executive staff, as well as a competent overall organization. However, he currently faces two major decisions that can have a major direct impact on the entire hospital and an indirect impact on its business standing within the community.

Delaware City Hospital is located in Delaware City, a mid-sized East Coast city (population 75,000) that has undergone a regional recession due to the relocation of three major local employers to the Sun Belt. Additionally, at the behest of the hospital's board of directors, DCH has recently absorbed three clinics (an additional 125 employees), which brings the hospital's full-time employee (FTE) count up to 825. It has also acquired a home for the aging that employs another 75 full-time employees. This total employee population of 900 is administered by a human resources staff of one executive and three managers.

The current vice-president of human resources, Richard Pierce, is slated for retirement next year, which gives the CEO approximately 18 months to select and prepare a successor. Because the organization prides itself on promoting from within, and because budget constraints preclude spending tens of thousands of dollars on an unwarranted executive search, the CEO will look to Pierce's staff for the next vice-president of human resources. However, Gale Avent, the senior manager of the staff, has removed herself from consideration due to her impending retirement in two years. Therefore, the CEO's first objective is to select either Michelle Newman, the current recruitment director, or Kevin O'Neill, the current director of training and development, for the position. The CEO's second objective is to implement a personnel development plan for the new vice-president, as well as one for the individual who does not get the job.

A set of files contains Pierce's personal notes and other information he has accumulated on the two candidates. The CEO studies these files and, in addition, makes his own notes on their abilities and proclivities. A review of the information, which the CEO collates under the general headings of "technical/professional," "managerial/supervisory," and "performance values," gives the CEO an idea of which candidate might be the better one given the current dynamics at DCH and in the customer community. Let's take a look at each candidate and determine first, based on the six specific headings on page 1 of figure 8-1 (p. 136), who is the better candidate.

□ The Candidates

Both candidates for the position of vice-president of human resources at Delaware City Hospital are competent and have proven valuable to the organization in their current roles. Unfortunately, only their performance evaluation forms from previous years, and notes that Richard Pierce has collected, are useful in assessing their promotability. As will be seen later in the chapter, the use of a personnel development plan would have greatly benefited this process. However, let's look at the existing data the CEO will consider now.

Kevin O'Neill

O'Neill has been with DCH for three years. During that time, he has completed an impressive array of projects and has achieved a high level of performance as director of training and development. He is a graduate of the University of Delaware, with a bachelor's degree in business administration. Currently, he is half-way through a graduate program, having attained 18 credits toward an MBA in human resources management. Prior to working for Delaware City Hospital, O'Neill worked in the pharmaceutical industry for four years, specifically in training and development. Training and development, then, is clearly the segment of human resources management that holds the most interest for him and where the majority of his contributions have been. At his previous position, O'Neill had no one reporting to him; at DCH he supervises two trainers and a secretary.

In considering O'Neill's strengths and weaknesses, there are many facets on the positive side of the ledger. He always thinks before acting and looks at both sides of an issue before making a decision. He feels a strong sense of allegiance with the local community and knows the particular nuances of Delaware City. He was born, raised, and still lives on Apple Street in downtown Delaware City, and thus has a broader frame of community reference than most of the managers in the organization. During his tenure at DCH, O'Neill has always attempted to learn as much as possible about managing human resources, as evidenced by his ability to fill in as compensation director during Gale Avent's one-month sick leave during the past reporting year. In managing the compensation function during this period, he learned a great deal about basic compensation systems and planned a particularly innovative compensation training program for first-line supervisors.

Away from the job, O'Neill participates actively in local community youth activities as an athletic coach and organizer. A former high school sports star, he works easily with youth, utilizes his training skills, and participates in sports as a natural avocation.

The CEO has noticed that, on a personal note, O'Neill is very direct and candid in discussions with both the CEO and members of the executive staff. However, from time to time the CEO has observed him use a different communication style with hourly employees, seeming less direct, a little more "accommodating," and perhaps not as genuine as he is in dealings with upper management. The CEO's opinion of this is simply that O'Neill, not as comfortable with the rank and file, perhaps wants to establish the fact that he is "one of them," just a "guy from Delaware City" who made it into management.

Because Pierce's background lacked training and development, O'Neill has had to set his own directions and objectives. This includes setting his goals each year, learning more about the training and development applications in health care, and learning generally about the health care business, knowledge that is so critical to the success of a vice-president of human resources. Whereas many of his training and development ideas and applications are from pharmaceutical industry models and systems he learned in that sector, O'Neill is constantly trying new ideas for all levels of management. He is particularly excited about the opportunity to provide training to the clinics and to newer employees, who have never been in an organization where training and development systems are part of the norm.

Figure 8-1.   Management Personnel Development Planning Form: Page 1

Name: _____ Position: _____ Date in Position: _____

Reviewing Manager/Executive: _____ Date: _____ Last Planning Date: _____

Technical/Professional Assets	Managerial/Supervisory Strengths	Strong Performance Values

Technical/Professional Liabilities	Managerial/Supervisory Weaknesses	Weak Performance Values

Figure 8-1. (Continued) Management Personnel Development Planning Form: Page 2

Name: _____ Promotability Range: _____

Performance Rating: _____ Short-/Long-Term Potential: 1. _____

Possible Successor: _____ 2. _____

Training and Development Plan   **Mentor Activities Plan**   **Progressive Action Plan**

General Comments

O'Neill is clearly a very dedicated individual. He has vacation days "backed up" from three years ago and has taken only one sick day during the entire three years. Furthermore, through reading and MBA coursework he has become somewhat of an "expert" on labor and collective bargaining. This is a particularly strong attribute, as Delaware City Hospital has in excess of 230 union members; also, several segments of the recently acquired clinics are unionized. O'Neill seems to have a natural interest in labor law and the collective-bargaining process. In summary, O'Neill's performance evaluation has indicated an ability to respond well to crises, to be an effective leader in the organization, and to complete all contracted objectives. This has come from a strong work ethic, a talent for adaptability, and a steadfast dedication to Delaware City Hospital, coupled with a natural interest in his job and its span of activities.

On the negative side of the ledger, O'Neill has a distinct proclivity for overenthusiasm for conducting training sessions, sometimes to the point of overlooking other required activities. As a result, his performance is uneven; it is usually stronger in areas having to do with training and development and employee relations and is somewhat lacking in the areas of compensation and basic personnel administration. Additionally, he has exceeded his budget several times in implementing new programs and introducing novel in-service programs. Furthermore, the implementation of these programs was not as timely as they should have been, which caused a lot of consternation and apprehension among senior management and the employees who would benefit from these programs.

A proverbial "grey area" exists in O'Neill's performance in dealing with other departments. For example, he served on the hospital community marketing committee but did not make a particularly strong contribution. This was disappointing to the CEO, who figured this assignment would take full advantage of O'Neill's community ties and apparent interest in community activities.

Another grey area example is O'Neill's questionable ability to conduct a management skills program for physician managers and directors. This was a key objective, something that certainly would raise the morale and motivation of the physician leaders in the hospital. The seminars were received as being "good but not great." Although O'Neill cannot be faulted completely, his performance in training and development in this case should have been stronger.

Overall, Kevin O'Neill would be a worthy candidate for the vice-president position. Clearly, his shortcomings can be developed and are certainly outweighed by his strengths. In high-visibility situations, such as his work on the employee relations committee and in his introduction of equal opportunity rights and nondiscrimination training, O'Neill has played a prominent part in the organizational development of Delaware City Hospital. However, he is not an automatic choice for the position.

Michelle Newman

Michelle Newman is equally qualified for the position, although she possesses a different set of skills and perhaps a different perspective on management of health care human resources. Newman is a graduate of the Delaware School of Nursing, with a bachelor of science degree. She is currently working on a master's in hospital administration from Delaware City State University, and in fact has completed 24 credits toward that degree.

Newman has worked at DCH for more than 11 years. Her initial employment was as a staff nurse, a position she held for six years. She then became a nurse recruiter, a position in which she produced uncommonly good results for two years. That led to her past three years as recruitment director, during which time she has performed at a superior level and done a particularly good job in recruiting technical employees and clinical staff. In her last two years as a staff nurse, Newman worked as a team leader, supervising up to eight nurses on two different shifts. Since moving to the human resources department, particularly in the past two years as recruitment director, she has supervised four employees, two recruiters, and two office/clerical personnel.

Newman is very dedicated to Delaware City Hospital, knows virtually everyone in the organization, and has stated that she hopes Delaware City Hospital will be her first, last, and only employer.

Newman learned a great deal about recruitment with guidance and instruction from Pierce, who was recruitment director prior to becoming vice-president of human resources. From becoming a particularly skilled recruiter and with Pierce's guidance, Newman has progressed steadily from nurse recruitment to recruitment of all types of hospital personnel at all levels. This broad-based ability has been augmented by her implementation of a systematic structured selection system for all areas of the organization. Furthermore, she has instituted turnover studies and exit interviews in critical areas of the organization, activities that save a great deal of time and money in both the recruiting and organizational development process. Furthermore, she has acquired demonstrative, useful experience in personnel reporting. In fact, she has implemented management information systems (MISs) for personnel administration and performance evaluation systems.

Away from the job, Newman is involved in local community activities, some of which are health-related, and in church activities in her hometown of Jacksonport, a small rural town 25 miles from Delaware City. Newman is very forthright in saying that she prefers the pace and activity of Jacksonport to Delaware City but enjoys the hospital activities and its particular culture.

Newman is perceived as a very good listener by all employees. Of particular note is her involvement with the Hispanic employees in the organization; they comprise 14 percent of the total hourly population of the DCH staff and 28 percent of the staff in the four new entities recently added to the hospital organization. In fact, she is very fluent in Spanish.

In terms of interpersonal skills, Newman always takes a very firm stance after making any decision, and she sticks with her conclusion and planned forms of action despite any counterarguments. From time to time, however, she is seen as being a little "hard-headed."

Newman was a prime player on the Delaware City Hospital community action committee. In addition, she coauthored, along with Gale Avent, the hospital's new affirmative action plan and equal opportunity policy.

All of her systems and approaches to human resources management are pretested and drawn from hospital environments, notably her recruitment, selection, and retention tactics. She is adept at utilizing agencies for recruitment of both computer and office clerical personnel. She has used school recruitment strategies for nurses, therapists, and skilled technicians. A combination of these strategies has been satisfactory and has allowed Delaware City Hospital to enjoy full staffing levels most of the time. Her last performance evaluation by Pierce indicated a 100 percent achievement of all objectives, and major cost savings on nurse and medical technician recruitment.

On the negative side of the ledger, Newman has a tendency to work closely only with nursing and other "traditional" job categories. Indeed, she is unfamiliar with marketing, finance, and other business departments—an outgrowth of her belief that in essence a hospital is not really a "business" like other businesses. She admits that she "has a problem" in referring to the hospital's patients as "customers."

On another note, Newman has stated openly that the recent acquisition of the new clinics and home for the aging was a "big mistake." This distaste for the business aspect of these facilities is evidenced in that, to date, she has not even visited these facilities, even though they are sorely in need of her services.

In the "grey area" category, Newman pursued several opportunities to educate herself about new performance evaluation systems. However, she passed up a great opportunity to attend seminars on employee relations and labor law.

Furthermore, although her reputation throughout the organization is that of someone who is very "bottom line" oriented, she is a major advocate of nursing and has vocally supported pay raises and benefit enhancement for nurses. This seems only natural, as she is a former nurse herself and feels nursing services carry a certain degree of importance as a major segment of the employee population.

☐ The Personnel Training and Development Plan

Although either of these candidates could certainly accomplish the mission of the vice-president of human resources, the CEO still needs to choose between the two. In an effort to be as objective as possible, he begins to draft a personnel training and development plan for each candidate.

A knowledgeable health care manager would take inventory of all physical assets and conduct an audit of all fiscal assets upon taking over a new position. Unfortunately, many times the most important resource—human resources—is not analyzed, inventoried, or audited. The CEO of Delaware City Hospital, as already demonstrated by his study of Richard Pierce's files and based on his own observations, has recognized that a personnel training and development plan could be used for this purpose.

The planning form he adopts is somewhat more complicated than the one in figure 7-2 because O'Neill and Newman are managers whose managerial/supervisory strengths need to be inventoried. The modified planning form in figure 8-1 can help meet a variety of objectives:

- The planning form extracts the most vital information from performance evaluations to provide the organization with a reference base for internal promotion considerations, transfers, and any other types of personnel moves among the management ranks.
- The form acts as a planning guide for both the manager and his or her direct managerial reports in a variety of essential performance categories.
- The form acts as a planning tool for departmental and organizational programs, as well as an instrument for determining "backups" and other long-range managerial staffing considerations.

Page 1 of this modified planning form contains a certain amount of administrative information. At the top is the employee's name and position. The employee's salary level could be added after the position. Next is the date that the employee started at the particular subject position, along with the reviewing manager/executive's name, the date that the planning form is being completed, and the last date that a planning form was executed.

Below this information is a space for listing the manager's technical/professional assets. This includes all of the employee's technical skills, business acumen, and other practical abilities on the job. Immediately below the assets is a space for listing any liabilities or shortcomings the employee may have with regard to his or her technical acumen that need to be addressed later through some sort of developmental activity.

The next column is entitled "managerial/supervisory strengths," with a space below for listing weaknesses. Managerial/supervisory strengths can include financial management skills—such as budget preparation or fiscal control—as well as planning, delegation, and performance evaluation skills. The entire range of interpersonal management skills should also be considered here, including communication, team development, conflict management, interviewing, and general employee relations. Other skills such as creativity, independent judgment, stress and time management, and other personal skills should also be evaluated as either a strength or a weakness.

The third column offers space for listing strong and weak performance values, such as those discussed in chapter 3 and in appendix A. Remembering that this form is simply a guide, the manager should simply identify the particular factor (such as "integrity") on the form, and on a separate page or in a manager's notebook list specific evidence that supports whether the value is a strength or a weakness. This not only helps to educate the employee, it also provides the proper reinforcement for strengthening the values that comprise the staff member's work personality.

On page 2 of the planning form, another set of administrative data should be filled out. This includes the most recent performance rating, which is taken strictly from the performance evaluation form, and a space to indicate who this individual's successor might be. In the right-hand corner, the form can include a space to indicate what position might be the next step in this individual's career if he or she were to be promoted immediately within the organization. Below this space are two spaces for recording other potential positions the individual would be qualified to fill over the short and long term.

Under the heading "training and development plan" on page 2 of figure 8-1, the CEO lists all activities that will help the personal development of the two candidates. (See figures 8-2 and 8-3 for specific information on this.) This would include seminars, in-service activities, and any other formal or informal educational activities. He has asked both candidates to participate actively in planning this section and to make as many suggestions as possible. Ideas besides seminars and other traditional forms of education, such as a reading list, understudy activities, and cross-training, are to be pursued.

The next section on page 2 of figure 8-1, "mentor activities plan," lists all activities in which the CEO and the candidates will participate on a one-on-one basis. Mentoring activities can include weekly meetings, or the candidate's assisting the CEO in a particular area, or the CEO's providing "point-specific" guidance in a particular technical or managerial area. Once again, the candidates' input has been encouraged, acknowledged, and accepted whenever possible; but the CEO has made sure to play a major role in setting up the mentor activities.

The CEO next uses the "progressive action plan" to indicate any personnel development strategies (appendix D), customer community strategies (appendix E), or any other strategies that might be used in the next year to both enhance employee development as well as maximize his or her contributions to the organization.

Finally, a section is provided for general comments to accommodate any remarks not specifically stated elsewhere in the planning form, or any plans that need to be enhanced through additional commentary. In figures 8-2 and 8-3 the CEO has indicated that he will pursue the development plan for each candidate immediately, and continue each plan once he has decided which candidate to promote.

☐ Case Analysis

More than 1,000 health care executives worked on this case study during their attendance at the author's various seminars. Perhaps not unexpectedly, there is usually a 50–50 split on who should get the job, for each candidate brings valuable experience and solid performance values to the vice-presidential position. It is the author's contention that the various viewpoints, perspectives, and proclivities of the seminar's participants shade their judgment in selecting the right candidate for the job.

What is clear, however, is that the use of a personnel development plan enables managers to make a sounder decision when promoting a manager. Richard Pierce was probably negligent in his responsibilities by not completing a personnel development plan for Newman and O'Neill. Furthermore, as a vice-president of human resources, he should have set a good example by using this planning system to develop the skills of his two direct reports. In addition, he should have instituted a personnel development planning system for all managers across the organization. If he had done so, not only would the CEO's decision be more clear-cut, but the organization would have had a smoother transition period during Pierce's pending retirement.

Of course, if both Newman and O'Neill are equally qualified, the CEO would have made a subjective decision anyway. However, this decision would need to be based on the specific needs of Delaware City

Hospital both now and in the future. If we assume that the future outlook of the hospital is to integrate the three clinics it recently acquired and to strengthen the organizational development programs, then O'Neill would be the proper choice. Conversely, if we assume that the home for the aging and its strong nursing populace, and the several personnel administrative responsibilities that go along with it, are to take precedence over training and development, then Newman would be the proper choice. In either case, the use of a personnel development plan would be most helpful 18 months from now when a decision has to be made.

Figure 8-2. Management Personnel Development Planning Form for Kevin O'Neill: Page 1

Name: _____Kevin O'Neill_____ Position: _____Director/T&D_____ Date in Position: ___2/88___

Reviewing Manager/Executive: ___R. Pierce/V.P., H.R.___ Date: _11/92_ Last Planning Date: _11/91_

Technical/Professional Assets	Managerial/Supervisory Strengths	Strong Performance Values
1. Training and development design and presentation	1. Conceptual and communication skills	1. Introspection
2. Employee relations skills	2. Crisis management	2. Compassion
3. Labor law and related systems	3. Consulting skills	3. Visibility
		4. Social awareness
		5. Customer commitment
		6. Allegiance

Technical/Professional Liabilities	Managerial/Supervisory Weaknesses	Weak Performance Values
1. Wage and compensation administration	1. Budgeting and fiscal management	1. Quality
2. Recruitment practices	2. Basic supervisory skills	2. Optimization of resources
3. Hourly employee training and development	3. Time management	3. Industry

☐ Practical Applications

The two-page planning form in figure 8-1 can be a strong organizational development tool. It acts as a conduit for much of the information in this book in that it provides the manager and his or her direct reports with a clear direction for developing skills and values. It also fosters participatory management and lends a strategic planning orientation to the human resources development process.

The following specific applications may help you apply the principles of personnel development planning to your own work setting:

Figure 8-2. (Continued) Management Personnel Development Planning Form for Kevin O'Neill: Page 2

Name: _____ Kevin O'Neill _____ Promotability Range: Vice-President, Human Resources

Performance Rating: 423 (of 500 max.) Short-/Long-Term Potential: 1. Director level

Possible Successor: _____ J. Smith _____ 2. Senior Vice-President

Training and Development Plan	Mentor Activities Plan	Progressive Action Plan
1. Intensive seminar in wage and compensation administration	1. Weekly "one-on-one" meetings with CEO	1. Implement organizationwide wage survey
2. Management skills training	2. Participate in board meetings with CEO	2. Institute training and development program for newly acquired facilities
3. Financial skills for the nonfinancial manager	3. Travel with CEO to state health care conference	
4. Reading list in labor relations		3. Organize open house for new employees at all facilities
5. Additional cross-training in benefits administration	4. Advise CEO on executive retreat content	4. Conduct attitude survey in all facilities

General Comments

Pursue established plan immediately and continue plan upon promotion to Vice-President, Human Resources (or upon promotion of other candidate). Review progress in three months.

Figure 8-3. Management Personnel Development Planning Form for Michelle Newman: Page 1

Name: ___Michelle Newman___ Position: ___Recruitment Director___ Date in Position: ___2/88___

Reviewing Manager/Executive: ___R. Pierce/V.P., H.R.___ Date: ___11/92___ Last Planning Date: ___11/91___

Technical/Professional Assets	Managerial/Supervisory Strengths	Strong Performance Values
1. Recruiting skills	1. Cost containment/ fiscal management	1. Knowledge
2. Nursing/medical staff support	2. Supervisory skills	2. Optimization of resources
3. Selection, personnel administration, and MIS in personnel arrangement	3. Planning skills and general organizational abilities	3. Compassion
		4. Dependability

Technical/Professional Liabilities	Managerial/Supervisory Weaknesses	Weak Performance Values
1. Employee relations and labor law	1. Knowledge of health care business areas outside human resources	1. Social awareness
2. Training and development systems and applications		2. Exemplary conduct
3. Comprehensive organizational development		3. Introspection
		4. Positive power
		5. Allegiance

1. Utilize the personnel development planning system with your reporting staff.
2. Explain the benefit and practical application of the planning system to your reporting supervisors and managers.
3. Utilize the case study to educate peers and staff members on the practical use of the planning system.
4. If you are a senior executive, encourage your human resources staff to implement a personnel development planning system throughout your organization.
5. Analyze the case again. Who would you select for vice-president if the organization was *your* place of employment?
6. Review the case with your reporting staff, with specific emphasis on the performance values evaluation.

Figure 8.3. (Continued) Management Personnel Development Planning Form for Michelle Newman: Page 2

Name: _____Michelle Newman_____   Promotability Range: _Vice-President, Human Resources_

Performance Rating: _417 (of 500 max.)_ Short-/Long-Term Potential: 1. _Director level_____

Possible Successor: ____A. Whitehead____   2. _Senior Vice-President_

Training and Development Plan	Mentor Activities Plan	Progressive Action Plan
1. Pursue coursework in employee relations and labor law	1. Accompany CEO on visits to new facilities	1. Implement criterion-based performance evaluation system
2. Cross-train in training and development area	2. Participate in board meetings with CEO	2. Institute training and development programs for newly acquired facilities
3. Work with marketing and public relations department	3. Accompany CEO to AHA annual convention	
4. Spend two days a week in first quarter at new facilities	4. Advise CEO on executive retreat content	3. Organize open house for new employees at all facilities
5. Attend seminar in basic health care business dynamics		4. Conduct attitude survey in all facilities

General Comments

Pursue established plan immediately and continue plan upon promotion to Vice-President, Human Resources (or upon promotion of other candidate). Review progress in three months.

7. Review the case study using blank planning forms. How and why would your assessment differ from the completed forms in figures 8-2 and 8-3?
8. Encourage your board of directors, if possible, to support the implementation of a personnel development planning system for their own review of executive management.
9. Combine the planning system with your current performance evaluation system.
10. Facilitate sessions with your staff in which they actively participate in the completion of their planning forms, and in setting a direction for the coming year.

Chapter 9

Progressive Business Strategies

To gain a measurable yield from a set of business norms, a health care organization must implement a series of progressive business strategies. These strategies should be focused in two basic areas: customer community strategies and organizational business strategies. *Customer community strategies* relate to those activities the organization can undertake to improve its presence in the community, its business acumen, and its image as a public trust. *Organizational business strategies* relate to specific programs the organization can undertake to increase its business effectiveness and, in the long run, its commercial success.

This chapter examines 10 major customer community strategies and 10 organizational business strategies. In each case, the author will review the strategy, how it was implemented by leading health care organizations, and how it can be implemented in your organization. The work sheets in appendix E can be used to plan specific applications to your organization and, more specifically, to craft goals for personnel development plans for managers (as described in chapter 8).

□ Customer Community Strategies

Any successful business (health care or otherwise) must recognize that the customer is at the top of the organizational chart. In the unique field of health care management, a successful administrator and his or her staff realize that the customer community—the geographic and demographic area the facility serves—is the paramount factor in the success equation. Therefore, it is vital for an administrator to strive constantly to implement progressive strategies relative to serving the customer community.

To be successful the organization must be perceived by the community as being an integral part of the community. This feeling of "ownership" underlies the community's support of the health care organization and the active participation in key health care–related activities by community members. Because most health care employees either are members or become members of the surrounding community, it is absolutely essential that the customer community be educated as to the overall mission, objectives, daily operations, and products and services offered by the health care organization.

Citizen Advisory Panels

A review of customer community strategies should begin with the interaction between citizens of the community and the health care facility. With this in mind, citizen advisory panels are becoming increasingly popular with many health care executives. In addition to tapping the expertise of the board of directors, many organizations rely on various citizen advisory panels to gather information about the community. Just as marketing firms use focus groups in designing and validating effective promotional tactics in key product components, many health care facilities now use citizen advisory panels for guidance on issues that affect the customer community and the organizations in the surrounding environment.

The formation of a citizen advisory panel is predicated on a need for detailed input on a specific issue of timely import to the facility. The responsibilities of a citizen advisory panel include attending meetings with members of the hospital's administration to discuss specific issues that affect current hospital practices and systems. These issues might include construction projects conducted by the hospital that affect local traffic, community-directed products and services, or the introduction of new health care services to the community. The meetings, monitored by various members of the staff, consist of a presentation of the underway issue or project and a question-and-answer component during which the citizens are polled for their reactions. The meetings should be well formatted in advance so as to reduce irrelevant dialogue, and the citizens should be rewarded in some small way—perhaps token jewelry or a savings bond—for their participation.

Citizen advisory panels are also excellent for gathering basic data on important short-term projects, that is, projects that are implemented according to a finite time sequence rather than on a continuing basis. Members of the management staff who will be involved with the project should be the key players and should present a specific agenda and set of objectives relative to the types of information they wish to elicit during the panel meetings.

Following are the advantages yielded by citizen advisory panels:

- Specific data relative to the project's implementation
- Community reactions prior to full implementation of the project
- Insights into various nuances of the project that might not be apparent to the health care organization but are very important to the customer community

Community Action Programs

Community action programs are projects the organization undertakes to help support significant social programs within the community. An example might be the support of a nonprofit venture such as homeless shelters or environmental cleanup efforts, or other more traditional community programs such as providing proper medical and ambulance support to the local high school athletic programs or at community fund-raisers.

An organization's marketing efforts are only as successful as their visibility within the customer community. Community action programs—the support of the health care organization to any high-profile, charitable undertakings or large-scale community activities—are excellent examples of opportunities that should be taken by the health care organization to increase its visibility and presence within the community.

Most U.S. and Canadian communities conduct programs such as walk-a-thons for various charities, newcomer programs, and other activities designed to help citizens become involved in meaningful causes as well as become acclimated to the community. For activities relative to community causes, it is recommended that the health care organization provide support by delegating the services of various members of the medical or ambulance staff to these causes. The hospital thus offers the community an operational resource in return for good advertising. In some cases, it might be useful for the organization to also donate its physical resources, such as its cafeteria meeting place, conference rooms, or educational facilities. If a health care organization is truly interested in being perceived as a public trust, its management and employees should make every effort possible to support community action programs and become involved as fully as possible.

Community action programs might also take the form of mobile health services units in which a wider spectrum of health care services can reach the community at strategic points. Examples include blood-mobiles, field-testing units, and helicopter or other airlift operations.

Community-Based Recruitment Programs

Considering that most of the organization's personnel, particularly non-exempt staff, come from the local community, a community-based recruitment program is essential. A program starts with announcements throughout the community of job openings at the organization. This includes posting notices on 3-by-5-inch index cards or on the organization's standard stationery in strategic locations—bulletin boards at supermarkets, cleaners, convenience stores, public libraries, and various places of worship. Doing so demonstrates a hospital's firm commitment to local hiring.

As with any recruitment strategy, it is essential that the hospital's recruitment staff ensure that all candidates' applications are reviewed judiciously and responded to appropriately. Recruiters should understand that if negative word-of-mouth publicity arises because the organization failed to respond appropriately, the entire community-based recruitment program could backfire and cause negative consequences to the hospital. A community-based recruitment program is a relatively inexpensive way of not only heightening the organization's visibility in the community, but also addressing the all-important dilemma of health care recruitment and the search for high-quality human resources.

Customer/Patient Feedback Systems

A successful business realizes that the crucial measure of its success is not how it compares with competitors but how it satisfies its customers. A wide array of methods should be devised to garner critical feedback, analyze it, and act on it. Such methods could include:

- Standard customer population survey instruments
- Targeted methods, such as exit interviews
- Visitor surveys, InfoCards, and hot-line numbers

The following sections explore three of these methods in more detail, beginning with the latter.

Consumer Hot Lines

A consumer hot-line number is a dedicated telephone line to the CEO/ administrator's office, available for consumers who have engaged the hospital's services. They can call to register complaints, offer suggestions, or otherwise comment on their experience with the facility. The consumer hot line can help the administration collect valuable information about the perceived needs and desires of the community, as well as elicit pertinent suggestions relative to hospital services and health care products. The use of a consumer hot-line number can also help the facility's marketing department in terms of gaining insights into how the health care organization is perceived within the community and relative to strategies that might be undertaken to optimize the organization's presence in the community.

From a quality standpoint, the number of complaints received versus the number of compliments received via a hot-line number can be instrumental in determining the overall quality of the organization as perceived by the community. Furthermore, comments can be quantified and keyed to specific departments. The consumer hot line does not necessarily have to be manned by a member of the staff. Rather, it can be answered by an answering machine whose tape is reviewed on a daily basis to ensure adequate and timely follow-up to complaints and other messages. Once again, for very little monetary expense, a health care organization can elicit a tremendous amount of potentially valuable information relative to quality of service, while demonstrating an awareness of and interest in the needs and desires of its customer community.

Customer Population Surveys

Another tool for determining customer/patient attitudes and gauging quality of service is the customer/patient survey. A well-designed survey instrument can be very beneficial in ascertaining the type of quality of service a customer/patient receives at the facility. Furthermore, it can help determine what word-of-mouth advertising the customer/patient might generate, as well as whether the respondent would use the organization's services in the future. Survey information can include opinions on the quality of medical service received, food service, visitors' services, and the facility in general.

Surveys also can yield any suggestions the customer/patient might have, and ways in which the organization might improve its service delivery. Survey design should take into account three basic principles of communication, namely:

1. A clear, easy-to-understand format of questions and answers
2. A format of no more than a total of 15 to 20 questions, because people become reluctant to fill out any form that is unnecessarily burdensome
3. Questions that have a direct intent and ask for specific comments and suggestions

The results of a customer/patient survey should be reviewed by all members of the administration, and survey results should be tabulated on a regular basis to identify significant trends and potential areas of positive or negative performance. The expense is very minimal in that the only expenses are for printing and mailing the forms. However, as in the case with many of these strategies, the yield and benefit can greatly outweigh the initial cost of implementation.

Visitor Surveys

In a similar vein, visitor surveys can be designed and distributed to individuals visiting patients at a health care organization. These forms can be distributed in the reception area or in other areas of easy access to visitors. Visitor surveys can yield useful information relative to parking, assistance rendered by various employees, and the visitor's perception of the patient's treatment. Surveys can be printed in such a manner that automatic mail return, paid by the sponsoring health care organization, is part of the form itself. This allows for easy completion and ensures that the form will be returned to the organization.

Visitor forms can also be returned via a suggestion box, which can be placed in the reception area. Forms can be stored on top of the box so that the visitor can complete the survey while waiting to see the patient, while waiting to receive information, or while waiting for visiting hours to commence. As is the case with customer/patient surveys, the visitor survey form should be easy to understand, have a set of specific directives and objectives, and be "short and sweet." Because the perception of a patient's family or friends might be directly related to a patient's perception of the hospital, results of visitor surveys should be given equal weight with the results of the customer/patient surveys in determining overall perceived quality and customer service of the institution.

Customer Service Award Programs

A visible means of supporting customer community interests is the establishment of a customer service award program. Within every health care organization, a system should be established to reward high commitment to customer/patient service past the normal compensation and benefits system. The establishment of such a system allows the organization to recognize premier service to customer/patients while citing examples of stellar community service for all members of the organization to emulate. The customer/patient service award can be part of the ongoing "employee of the month" program or be a separate award given at a special time. In addition to just presenting an award, the exact episode or set of circumstances that gave rise to the reward should be cited and publicized effectively throughout the organization.

The award should be something that provides enough of an incentive that the entire organization understands fully the importance attached to stellar customer/patient service. Because it is a terrific motivator, money might be a suitable reward, as might additional vacation days or a savings bond. Although many health care organizations stress the need for proactive customer service, very few seem truly committed to this ideal of putting the customer at the top of the organizational chart. The installation of a customer service reward program would emphasize putting the patient first.

Health Information Publications

The distribution of health information publications is one way organizations can provide essential information to their customer communities on a timely basis. For example, health information pamphlets could describe a particular malady affecting a large segment of the population (such as AIDS) or one of notable interest to the customer community (a flu epidemic). In publicizing such information, preventive measures should be explained, symptoms detailed, and perhaps most important, directions given on where and how to contact qualified personnel at the health care organization. These publications should then be placed at strategic areas throughout the customer community—libraries, post offices, and other high-traffic places.

A good integrated publications strategy might be to ask individual community members, using customer/patient surveys, what prominent issues are of interest to them and to use their responses as a basis for the type of information publication to be disseminated. By undertaking a health information publications program, the organization not only provides a necessary community service, it also presents itself as the expert in the particular subject area, as well as the main provider to combat the affliction described.

Drug Awareness Programs

A specific area of interest to every community in North America is drug awareness. With the widespread usage of illegal drugs, organizations in the public and private sector are trying to provide information on drug abuse and its consequences.

Health care organizations have an opportunity not only to maximize their credibility within the community but also to live up to their responsibility as a public trust by instituting drug awareness programs. These can include conducting drug awareness seminars on-site as well as at local schools, cosponsoring drug awareness programs with the local police force and other public trusts within the community, and publishing pamphlets on drug use and addiction.

Drug awareness programs demonstrate clearly a facility's natural commitment to the health of its community. Because many hospitals and other health care organizations have drug treatment facilities, promoting awareness programs can be seen as an opportunistic or callous marketing strategy. But when one considers the scope of the drug problem and the scarcity of treatment facilities, these programs are a progressive business strategy as well as a community service.

One-Day Outpatient Programs

With increased competition coming from alternative health care delivery systems, such as HMOs, more traditional health care organizations have had to increase the scope and quantity of their one-day outpatient programs. Although services such as abortion are highly controversial, other services such as weight reduction programs and stress management programs have become part of ongoing outpatient programs.

Furthermore, routine blood tests and other short-term medical procedures have become part of the outpatient program in many progressive health care organizations. In fact, many organizations are establishing "day clinics," in which such procedures can be provided and managed in a short time period, and allow a community member access to high-quality medical and health care expertise on a reduced-cost basis. This not only provides necessary services on a timely basis, it also establishes the health care organization as a logical provider of all health care services the community member might need.

School Liaison Programs

School liaison and student employment are two features of a progressive approach to health care management that have been overlooked in recent times. With the end of the baby boom, the need for more entry-level workers within all ranks of an organization has become more critical than ever. To boost nursing school enrollments, as well as the general ranks of nonexempt employees, hospitals and other health care organizations must become more aggressive in their recruitment efforts.

Therefore, school liaison programs are extremely important. School liaison programs incorporate the presentation of critical-subject seminars to various local schools on a regular basis. Subjects range from drugs to birth control and other topics of importance to a teenager. These programs can also be augmented by presentations at "career days" at local high schools or junior colleges, where the local health care organization presents information on health careers and answers questions from students who might be interested in a career in health care. A secondary benefit is increased visibility for the health care organization, but the primary benefit of such an approach is that the organization can attract potential job applicants.

A follow-up to such programs is student employment, which can include internships and summer jobs that call for little or no expertise — maintenance positions, for example. In providing such jobs to the community, the organization is perceived as being interested in the community's youth. Also, the facility is grooming prospective (long-term) health care professionals. Traditional programs in this area, notably the candy stripers program in the nursing profession, have had time-honored success within the health care industry. As the scramble for qualified health care professionals at all levels becomes more intense, these strategies will become even more important to various health care organizations.

Employee Communication

Having good employee communication, as described in an earlier chapter, is another progressive customer community strategy, and the final strategy of this section of the discussion. Because most employees are members of the community, it is vital that managers maintain an "open-ear" program in addition to an "open-door" policy of management. An open-ear program basically entails listening closely to the perceptions of employees and the experiences relayed to them by their neighbors within the community. For example, in a small town most members of the community know if one of their neighbors is a hospital or health care worker and will invariably share their perceptions on treatment and quality. If these comments are properly relayed to the manager and shared throughout the organization, the organization can develop a very informal but infallible checks-and-balances system of ascertaining their perception within their customer community.

No matter what method or methods are used by a progressive health care organization, it is essential to recognize the need for collecting as much information as possible from the customer community and capitalizing on that information to provide better service over the course of time. In doing so, the organization not only establishes itself as a public trust but also as a progressive organization in every sense of the term.

☐ Organizational Business Strategies

In addition to taking progressive action to better serve its customer community, the organization must look at the strategies inherent in the conduct of its business. An assortment of business strategies — policies, programs, and systems to maximize performance — must be adhered to and pursued relentlessly if a health care organization is to remain successful.

Board Composition

A logical starting place for organizing business strategies is at the top, with the executive leadership, and, more specifically, with the composition of the board of trustees overseeing the services of the health care organization. The composition of a board of trustees is extremely important because the board is the main governing body of the organization and hence influences its objectives, goals, and directions. A board of trustees that understands the health care business, the community, and sound business practices in general is likely to be a great ally in the pursuit of excellence. On the other hand, a board of trustees locked into obsolete thinking about the health care business or preoccupied with strategies relative to non–health care businesses is likely to be a major hindrance to the pursuit of excellence and in some documented cases has caused the demise of health care organizations. Therefore, a progressive organization must review the composition of its board and ensure that members are all aware of current health care dynamics, sound business strategy, community needs and demands, and the direction and planning of a successful organization.

A logical composition for a board of trustees is the inclusion of members from three distinct groups. The first group should be individuals from local businesses who understand the local community, the dynamics of the community's structure, and the precepts of business success within that community. Local business leaders might include:

- Regional industry executives
- Finance/banking executives
- Successful entrepreneurs
- Local directors of national firms
- Large retailers
- Executives of major employers

The second group should be made up of individuals from the health care business who know the dynamics of the current health care environment and the state of change in which the profession is operating currently, and who have specific perceptions about succeeding in the health care field in these turbulent times. Health care business leaders include:

- CEOs of other, noncompetitive health care institutions
- Prominent physicians
- Directors of major nonprofit health care institutions
- Noted academics in health care
- Nonmilitant guild or union leaders
- Ancillary group leaders

The third group should consist of members of prominent community organizations such as local politicians and workers at other community-based organizations. These individuals can be vital in providing advice in various legal and political endeavors, as well as contributing guidance relative to issues relating to local economics, sociological composition, and other essential dynamics of community-based business. Local community leaders include:

- Elected public officials
- Major social leaders
- Civic action leaders
- Noted attorneys
- Noted academic leaders
- State/federal officials

All members of the board of trustees should share the same business norms and basic objectives as the health care administrator. There should be a distinct commitment not only to the customer but to the values of forthright tactics, high-quality service, social awareness, and perhaps most important, a commitment to the professional liberty of the health care administrator and his or her staff.

Departmental Planning

Once a set of organizational directives has been articulated by the health care administrator and endorsed by the board of trustees, a round of departmental "mission-relevant" planning sessions should occur. Each department head should submit to the supervising manager a set of objectives and actions to be undertaken in a given operational period to support the facility's mission and objectives. The reviewing manager in turn should review these goals and objectives, suggest additional actions, and customize each goal relative to attaining synergy among all reporting departments. In this fashion, all internal operations can be directed toward the facility's overall mission, objectives, and goals.

Strategic Planning

Armed with each department's "mission-relevant" plans, the administrator or CEO should conduct an executive strategic planning retreat. This retreat should be held at a location away from the facility, ideally at a conference retreat center or other location that will allow a certain degree of isolation away from beepers and phone calls. At these sessions, the CEO should recapitulate the departmental plans established for the organization and review the individual action plans submitted by the reporting managers. Furthermore, the CEO should challenge each staff member as to the meaningful application of each of the goals submitted—as well as the performance levels and potential of every manager and supervisor within the organization—and strive to establish a strategic plan for the next three years of operation. In establishing such a plan, more than group goals and specific organizational objectives should be reviewed: Also of prime importance are the organization's overall mission and factors that might challenge the organization's effectiveness, such as significant changes in the community or new or impending competition. These and other essential dynamics of the business environment should be discussed frankly and in the interest of providing tangible solutions for progressive action.

Monthly Meetings

The strategic planning retreat should be reinforced with a monthly staff meeting among the organization's executive group and monthly meetings with each department manager and his or her staff. One attribute of a meeting of this nature would be the inclusion of an interdepartmental "show-and-tell" component. That is, each staff member is invited to take a turn displaying new projects and relating other activities his or her department is pursuing that might interest other members of the organization. This not only helps to hone the staff's presentation skills, but it also promulgates information relative to operations throughout the organization and allows the opportunity for pertinent staff feedback and suggestions for maximizing the facility's performance.

Matrix Management

A by-product of these monthly meetings might be the establishment of a matrix management scheme. Two types of matrix management are the new project team and the mission-objective team.

The *new project team* incorporates the talents of managers and qualified personnel from two or more distinct departments working toward a common goal. An example of a new project team is a group of nursing supervisors working with several members of the personnel department to determine a new incentive-based performance evaluation system for nursing personnel, or perhaps to develop an alternative nursing recruitment program. Another example is the hospital pharmacist working with the security staff to ensure that all pharmaceuticals in the facility are secured safely. Larger projects that might be undertaken by a new project team include construction of a new wing or parking facility.

The *mission-objective team* meets the needs of atypical challenges and special circumstances. A mission-objective team brings together persons with specific technical expertise, managerial acumen, and an assortment of other educated perspectives from across the organization. The creative application of various executive and managerial talent by the mission-objective team can be invaluable to the organization in solving problems, resolving conflicts, establishing goals, and planning courses of action. Examples of mission-objective teams are review committees for employee benefits, crisis management teams, budget review teams, and discipline review teams or conflict mentors.

A benefit of establishing some form of matrix management is that the entire management team becomes more cohesive as members become more familiar with each other, and individual managers increase their scope of understanding and their spectrum of expertise by being exposed to other areas of the health care operation and thus strengthening the facility's overall know-how.

Community Executive Action

An organizational business strategy does not necessarily have to be a new or novel approach. It can be the enhancement of a normal activity that, in the day-to-day activities of a health care administrator, might be overlooked but is nevertheless essential toward maintaining good relations between institution and community. For example, most health care executives find the time in their busy schedules to participate in community activities that heighten the visibility of their organization as well as provide insight into the needs and demands of the community. Furthermore, these activities encourage the involvement of other members of the organization in the community, thus strengthening the organization's overall credibility.

To cite another example, many health care administrators are members of local Rotary Clubs and other service-oriented organizations within the community. This helps administrators understand the community better and formulate mission-oriented actions for the organization.

Some administrators are involved in local community politics. They might hold an elected office or participate consistently in the political life of their community. Their involvement, as well as that of their reporting staff, increases the administration's understanding of customer/ community needs and desires. Perhaps more important, political involvement helps integrate the goals and objectives of the community at large with the mission of the health care organization. As long as conflict of interest or eminent controversy is not part of the package, political involvement can provide numerous benefits for the participative manager and his or her organization.

Mission Achievement Committees

In a similar vein, the establishment of a mission achievement committee is a good strategy to ensure compliance and support of mission objectives by employees at every level of the health care organization. Mission achievement committees are composed of selected hourly and nonexempt employees throughout the health care organization's work force who meet regularly with the administrator and discuss ways in which the mission of the organization should be enhanced, defined, and reflected by the organization's daily actions.

Mission achievement committee members can suggest new programs the organization can undertake, as well as communicate ideas suggested to them by community members, in order to contribute to the formulation of the organization's business goals and directives. Furthermore, the involvement of committee members in local community activities can position them to reinforce perceptions gathered through citizen advisory panels and the various customer/patient feedback systems.

Organizational Advantage Programs

Successful health care organizations not only seek to constantly upgrade their operations, they seek opportunities to present programs and services that emphasize the organization's commitment to high-quality health care service. It is the duty of the organization's executive staff, in conjunction with all employees, to identify and present opportunities for these upgrades. Such opportunities are often first identified in quality enhancement (or similarly named) committees within the organization.

One such opportunity for upgrading services to employees is the implementation of intergenerational day-care services. Under such a program, residents of a home for the aging affiliated with the health care organization help to provide day care for the children of employees and medical staff personnel.

Another opportunity is the control of traffic in and out of the organization's physical plant. This often includes the reallocation of parking spots to help employees park their cars close to their workstations. New approaches to parking and traffic control can decrease employee stress and help to demonstrate the organization's commitment to helping its employees provide stellar health care services at all times.

Open-House Programs

Holding an open house is another way business norms can be enhanced and publicized not only to the customer community but to all staff members of a health care organization. Open houses are used primarily as a recruiting tactic but are also very important in increasing the understanding among the families of current employees as to the specific demands of the health care arena and what their family member goes through in any given day at work. Open houses should be conducted at least yearly by all health care organizations; publicized through the local media; and open to all members of the community, notably the families and friends of employees.

By having an opportunity to see where employees work, their family or friends will have a heightened awareness of and appreciation for that individual's job. Furthermore, family or friends might provide input as to the conduct of the organization's business and its "way of doing things." Finally, open-house programs enhance a facility's visibility in the community and facilitate potential recruitment.

Organizational Communication Tactics

The health care executive who does not take a proactive role in managing the media and press relations can be victimized by stories or reports that generate negative publicity for the organization. A facility's employee newsletter and its community-oriented publications are devices the executive can use to ensure that positive publicity is generated about the organization. By using an integrated strategy of asking mission achievement committees and other employees at all levels for interesting stories, insights, or episodes, the hospital's community relations department or (in a small organization) the health care executive, can generate "positive press" for use by the external media. This helps the esprit de corps of the organization, helps convince the public of its commitment to quality and customer service, and helps reemphasize a commitment to progressive health care management within the facility itself.

□ Practical Applications

The use of progressive health care business strategies is essential for any value-driven health care organization to flourish. The utilization of such strategies ensures proper community support and galvanization of all components of the organization. Having a corporate culture that supports value-driven performance is one thing; it is essential to also have a set of strategies that make commitment to value-driven performance a daily reality.

The following practical applications can help ensure that your organization has made more than a "lip-service" commitment to high-quality performance within the ever-changing health care business arena.

1. Review the business strategies discussed in this chapter for potential implementation in your area of responsibility.
2. Assess which strategies can be implemented in your organization in the short term.

3. Determine which strategies could be implemented in your organization over the long term.
4. Discuss certain strategies with the individual who manages the
   related function in your organization.
5. Review the specific strategies in appendix E for ideas on specific
   applications at your facility.
6. Garner the input of your direct reports in determining which strategy
   has the most potential for improving the performance of your particular area.
7. Add specific applications, based on your organization's needs, to the
   roster of strategies discussed in the text.
8. Discuss these strategies with your senior management and board
   for organizationwide implementation.
9. Use the strategies as part of your management retreat discussions.
10. Incorporate the strategies as discussion points for potential imple-
    mentation during strategic planning sessions.

Chapter 10

Case Study: Progressive Health Care Management

The essence of a value-driven health care organization is its ability to combine the ethical management principles described in this book with progressive approaches to health care management. In order to provide a complete illustration of this effective combination, the following case study has been constructed on several precepts of ethical management and numerous management strategies utilized by leading health care organizations.

The case study can provide three major benefits to the reader. First, it is a review of the major principles and strategies depicted in this book. Second, it provides a "cause and benefit" illustration of progressive management strategies in action. Finally, it can yield realistic insight into implementing several of these progressive management strategies into a specific organization.

☐ The Maryville Organization

Maryville Community Hospital (MCH) is a medium-sized facility located in the northwestern part of the United States. It was founded in 1934 largely as a not-for-profit entity to serve the needs of several small communities, which had sprouted as a direct result of the growing logging and railroad industries of the region.

The original board of directors represented a cross section of the area's civic and business leaders. The president and vice-president of the major railroad company and the two directors of the preeminent logging firm were represented, as were the school superintendent, two city councilmen from the area's two largest cities, and three members of local religious and social action groups. Figure 10-1 depicts the board membership at the hospital's origin, and figure 10-2 depicts membership in 1990. In both cases, no special-interest groups were catered to; nor were any "hidden agendas" represented by the constituency of the boards. The major objective of the board, in 1934 as well as in 1990, was to direct a progressive health care organization that would provide high-quality care to all needy members of the surrounding communities.

Following World War II, the area further developed when a major aircraft corporation built a plant in the Maryville area. This marked the beginning of a population explosion, which was further augmented by a real estate boom market due to a migration of northern-bound Californians looking for a less congested life-style. In the 1960s, the Mega-Tech Corporation, whose founders were Maryville residents, invented a sophisticated microchip that drew even more people to the area and increased the demand for Maryville health care services. By 1970, two other hospitals had established operations in the area: Central Community Hospital, which was located 10 miles east of Maryville, and Northern Oaks

Figure 10-1. Maryville Community Hospital Board of Directors (1934)

Name	Title/Organization	Board Position
Floyd Stevens	City Councilman/Belle Vista	Chairman
Leo Dunedin	President/Lewis Logging Company	Vice-Chairman
Davis Samuels	President/Purple Valley Railroad Company	Chairman
Jane Wilson	Director/Northwest Charities	Vice-Chairman
Debra Richman	Superintendent/Douglas County School System	Member
Joseph Ellis	Vice-President/Purple Valley Railroad Company	Member
Edna Graham	Director/Northwest Red Cross	Member
Fred Liston	City Councilman/Oak City	Member
Lynn McGraw	Chief Financial Officer/Lewis Logging Company	Member
James Hartley	President/AFL-CIO Local #816	Member

Figure 10-2. Maryville Community Healthcare Corporation Board of Directors (1990)

Name	Title/Organization	Board Position
Nick Bonavena	President/Mega-Tech	Chairman
Manny Davis	President/Linial Aircraft	Vice-Chairman
Norma Bates	Mayor/Belle Vista	Vice-Chairman
Fred Liston	Mayor/Oak City	Vice-Chairman
Ellen Graham	Director/Northwest Red Cross	Member
Ben Como	President/Chico Grande Real Estate	Member
Roger Dixon	Superintendent/Douglas County Schools	Member
Marla Santana	President/Technical Workers Union	Member
David Samuels, Jr.	President/Purple Valley Railroad	Member
Janet McGraw-Grant	CEO/Lewis Logging	Member

Hospital, a venture capital–financed institution located 10 miles to the north of MCH. Although the demographics of a booming population and increased demand for services was in MCH's favor, the increased competition from these two new entities provided a formidable challenge to its growth and development.

Upon the retirement of MCH's long-tenured administrator in 1972, the board conducted an extensive search for a new CEO/administrator. Recruitment efforts included using the referral networks provided by several national health care organizations, advertising in several prominent health care management journals, and using board contacts throughout the industry at large to elicit a wide-ranging list of prospective candidates. After considering more than 100 resumés, the board "short-listed" a roster of five finalists who were flown to Belle Vista, the largest town in Maryville's area and the site of the facility itself. From this list, two finalists were selected. One finalist declined the initial salary range advertised by the Maryville board and told the board that he would not consider the position unless the salary range was raised by $15,000 per year. The other finalist, satisfied with the salary range, was invited to Belle Vista for a final meeting with the Maryville board. This candidate, Marty Fontana, was encouraged to bring his wife and children along to visit the area and meet with some real estate representatives the board had arranged to conduct a tour of the area and show potential housing. This family-oriented trip was part of the board's strategy to ensure not only that the new administrator was comfortable with the job position, but that his family was comfortable with the living conditions, life-style, and school system in the Maryville community. By meeting this objective, they were not only attracting a long-term administrator to their facility, they were also making sure that a "true match" was made between the key executive, the organization, and the community it serviced.

Immediately after taking the position, Marty Fontana submitted five major objectives to the board that represented essential organizational objectives and important business goals for the Maryville organization. The board in turn added three objectives to the list, for a total of eight bonus-eligible objectives, which Fontana would pursue in his initial year as the MCH CEO. These objectives were prioritized, the most important being given a 40 percent weighted value—the acquisition of a nursing home that would provide long-term Maryville customer/patients with a residential care option for their golden years. As many of the logging and railroad company veterans reached retirement, the need for such a facility was paramount and in keeping with the Maryville business objective of providing high-quality health care to all community members. This also represented a continuation of growth for Maryville Community Hospital, which by now had grown to approximately 275 beds and close to 800 employees.

Other objectives for Marty Fontana's first year included the establishment of a five-year strategic plan, successful management of a minor
expansion program in the east wing of the hospital, the establishment
of tighter financial controls for the entire organization, and an expansion plan for medical services in several specific areas. Each of the goals
was rewritten by Fontana and approved by the board to contain specific
deadlines, financial parameters, and representations of numbers and percentages for each goal. Several of these goals — in fact the majority of
them — were later incorporated into the five-year plan. For example, the
tighter fiscal controls would evolve over the next five years as a constant
theme in the goals of all the organization's executives and the plan
provided benefits to the organization such as bonuses for cost-saving
suggestions, a new computerized accounting system, and a better internal auditing system of all Maryville expenditures.

The expansion of Maryville Community Hospital as a total health care
service organization began with the purchase of the Golden Isles Retirement Center. Golden Isles was a well-run facility that was established in
1952 in a resort area 15 miles south of MCH. Its owner, Gene Silver, was
looking forward to retiring in three years. Fontana negotiated not only a
purchase agreement with Silver, but also a two-year management contract in which Silver would run the facility as a paid executive of Maryville
Community Hospital. Fontana set a series of goals and objectives for Silver
to meet in each of these two years, all of which suggested a direction toward
not only the continuance of stellar organizational performance but also
a plan of action for assimilating the retirement center into the greater
Maryville organization. Fontana based his decision to purchase this facility primarily on the ethical principles and "customer- first" philosophy
that Silver had used in his management and leadership of the facility.

Maryville expanded further in 1984 when it bought the West Park
Rehabilitation Center. This facility, also located within a 15-mile radius
of Maryville's home community of Belle Vista, was a well-known rehabilitation center established primarily with funds provided from the railroad and logging union workers' pension investment fund. The facility
needed finances to maintain its high-quality operation and to purchase
state-of-the-art equipment as the union funds dwindled due to shrinking membership. By eliciting a large financial commitment from the
Mega-Tech Corporation and the aircraft manufacturer, Fontana was able
to purchase and revitalize the facility. Its new name became the Maryville
Rehabilitation Center, and in the same year the Golden Isles Retirement
Center became the Maryville Retirement Center. As he explained to the
board, Fontana's rationale for the name change was that Maryville had
a good, time-honored name within its customer community, which from
a marketing viewpoint would benefit these new additions while instill-
ing a sense of "family" to all members of all three organizations.

The Board of Directors

As figures 10-1 and 10-2 reflect, the 1990 board of directors is very similar in size and composition to the original 1934 board. The chairman of the board, Nick Bonavena, is the president of the largest employer in the Belle Vista–Oak City area and also the president of MCH's biggest financial benefactor. The corporation's second-largest benefactor, Linial Aircraft, is represented by its president, and the remaining two vice-chairman positions are filled by the mayors of the organization's two largest customer communities. The other members are drawn from a historically validated mix of community and civic action leaders, a school superintendent, and other community industries. This board meets once a month formally and lends specific expertise in the areas of fund-raising, strategic direction, and fiscal planning.

At Marty Fontana's request, individual members of the board contribute specific expertise and resources to the Maryville Community Healthcare (MCH) mission. For example, all of the computer and MISs in all three Maryville facilities are either Mega-Tech products or equipment that is compatible with Mega-Tech products and donated by that organization. A second example: When additional parking spaces were needed for both medical staff and visitors to the main hospital facility in Belle Vista, Ben Como of Chico Grande Real Estate secured a favorable deal for some land strategically adjacent to the facility.

A third example of this true partnership is evidenced in the hospital's biannual outings on the Purple Valley Railroad, which is now largely a tourist railroad. Every six months, all employees and their families are invited to go on a railway outing from Belle Vista through Oak City, and on to a large state park. After a company picnic at this state park, all of the employees are then returned to their home communities via the excursion railroad. This not only helps morale, it serves as a model promotional effort by the railroad in obtaining other corporate clients.

A fourth example is evidenced by the participation of Roger Dixon, Douglas County's superintendent of schools, with the training and development specialist and employee relations managers who work for Joe Tunney, Maryville Community Healthcare's CEO. In an effort to provide the non–high school graduates of the entire Maryville system with an opportunity to obtain their GED, the Douglas County school system sponsors GED preparation courses at each of the three health care facilities in time slots that are compatible with normal working hours and irregular shifts. By bringing this opportunity to the facilities, the interested workers enjoy a sense of convenience and commitment from both the organization and the school system in obtaining this all-important credential. It shows a sense of sincere interest in the employees' development, as well as provides the hospital, rehabilitation center, and retirement center with a better-qualified work force. In a similar fashion, the Douglas County school system also provides an array of courses in typing, technical areas, and other skills that contribute to hourly employee development.

Furthermore, the Douglas County Community College has recently instituted a series of entry-level college courses for the continued development of the Maryville Community Healthcare Corporation's GED graduates. Fontana goes to great lengths to sponsor a graduation ceremony and other recognition programs to acknowledge the accomplishments of these adult scholars.

Other examples of board–organization cooperation have occurred within levels of management. Many operations specialists of Linial Aircraft have donated their time to upgrading the logistics programs of all three facilities. Norma Bates, the mayor of Belle Vista, and Fred Liston, the second-generation politician from Oak City, have assisted the hospital in a variety of ways relative to political and social issues, for example, filing of taxes and affirmative action programs. By working hand in hand with these government agencies, Fontana's organization ensures that any emergent problems are dealt with proactively and correctly before they become an administrative headache.

☐ The Executive Staff

Fontana inherited a relatively strong staff at the commencement of his tenure as CEO of Maryville Community Hospital, and over the years has built a strong current lineup of executives and managers throughout the corporation. His own staff consists of five direct reports (shown in figure 10-3), whom he formally calls his "management committee." Fontana believes strongly in a maximum of five direct reports, with seven as an absolute maximum. This belief is based on his experience in organizations with other management structures he has deemed ineffective. With a group of five, Fontana feels as though major decisions affecting the entire corporation can be discussed and analyzed and solutions planned with a broad-based perspective. A hidden advantage in having five direct reports is that Fontana never has to act as a "tiebreaker" on critical matters requiring a quorum. In a similar vein, he is pleased that the board has nine members so Bonavena, as the tenth member and chairman, can similarly act as a leader without having to cast a tie-breaking vote.

Members of Fontana's management council are all well versed in health care, specific technical knowledge, and most important, the art, science, and skills of general management. Cynthia Rose, director of the Maryville Retirement Center, learned her craft during her 14 years in the homes for the aging industry, the last 7 of which as Gene Silver's chief

Figure 10-3. Organizational Chart for Maryville Community Healthcare Corporation

Marty Fontana
President
Maryville Community Healthcare Corporation (MCHC)

Cynthia Rose
Director
Maryville Retirement Center

Operations and financial functions of Maryville Retirement Center

James Black
Administrator
Maryville Community Hospital

Operations and financial functions of Maryville Community Hospital and Maryville Rehabilitation Center

Harry Tyson
CFO
Maryville Community Healthcare Corporation

All financial, accounting, and management information systems functions of Maryville Community Healthcare Corporation

Helen Clay
COO
Maryville Community Healthcare Corporation

All operations, marketing, and patient relations functions of Maryville Community Healthcare Corporation

Joe Tunney
CAO
Maryville Community Healthcare Corporation

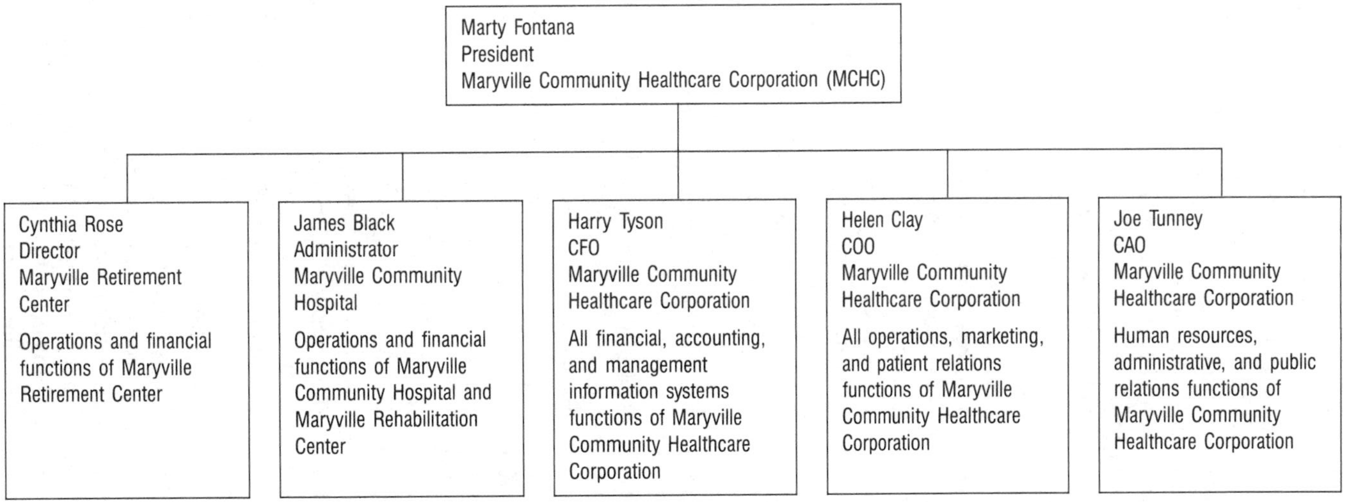

Human resources, administrative, and public relations functions of Maryville Community Healthcare Corporation

assistant administrator at what was then known as Golden Isles Retirement Center. When Fontana investigated possible retirement homes for acquisition, Rose's strength as a manager and potential director of the facility was one of the major contributing factors to his decision. Part of Silver's two-year employment contract, and a major contingent factor of the purchase itself, was Silver's assisting Rose in all aspects of operational management and educating her in specific areas of the operational and fiscal management of the facility, which would prove critical once under the Maryville umbrella. Rose was academically well prepared for her position, possessing a bachelor's degree in business administration from the state university and a master's in health administration, for which she wrote a thesis titled "Financial Management of Retirement Centers." In addition to her responsibilities as director of the Maryville Retirement Center, Rose is on the board of directors of Northwest Charities and is vice-chairman of Douglas County's Special Olympics Program. Furthermore, she is on the state advisory board for retirement issues, and an active member and officer in the National Association of Nursing Home Administrators. This organization encompasses members in the retirement center business, as well as those facilities with customer/residents with special needs.

James Black is the administrator of Maryville Community Hospital. After the retirement of Fontana's original vice-president of operations in 1972, Fontana recruited Black from his native Minneapolis to work as his vice-president of operations in Belle Vista. Fontana himself had come from Minnesota to the Maryville job and knew of Black peripherally based on his experience in the Twin Cities. However, Fontana garnered an impressive body of references on Black and, in addition to interviewing him personally, had Black interview with the board and with other members of the executive management team with whom he would be working.

Black has a bachelor's and master's in business administration, and has worked in health care for 15 years including his time at Maryville. Previous positions have included department head at a large Minnesota hospital, assistant administrator of operations at the same facility, and director of operations at Maryville. Black is an elected member of the school board and is extremely active with youth athletics throughout the Douglas County area.

Fontana presented an initial objective to Black of spearheading the purchase of Maryville (formerly West Park) Rehabilitation Center. By including Black in any decisions and letting him learn a great deal about the facility, a natural transition occurred later. Black was given control over managing this facility along with MCH as the organization evolved and Fontana removed himself as hospital administrator to become president of the entire Maryville Community Healthcare Corporation.

Harry Tyson is the chief financial officer (CFO) of the Maryville Community Healthcare Corporation. Possessing a master's degree in finance and accounting from a top East Coast college, Tyson was a junior partner for a major national accounting firm, which was employed by the state government to run a special audit of all hospitals receiving large amounts of government aid. Fontana was so impressed with Tyson's diligence and hard work that he kept tabs on him as he progressed within the accounting organization, and then as finance director at a small HMO corporation. When Fontana's financial director retired prior to the acquisition of West Park Rehabilitation Center and the complete assimilation of Golden Isles Retirement Center, Fontana brought Tyson in for a round of comprehensive interviews and ultimately hired him as the CFO of the new organization. Tyson is the youngest member of the management council, but perhaps the most active in community organizations. He is the coach of a state championship youth hockey team, teaches continuing education courses in finance, and provides annual tax return seminars to MCH employees as part of the employee assistance program.

Helen Clay is the chief operating officer (COO) of the Maryville Community Healthcare Corporation. The longest-tenured member of the management team, Clay started her career at MCH in 1967 as a nurse. She progressed rapidly through the nursing hierarchy while working at night on a master's in health administration at the University of the Northwest. She was the second candidate of choice when Black was hired as vice-president of operations, failing to get that position because she lacked experience in nonnursing operations. However, Fontana offered her the opportunity of becoming Black's successor if she mastered the tenets of operational management. Clay pursued this development plan with a vengeance; she designed a marketing plan for the organization and pursued every opportunity to learn as much as possible about the emergent facet of patient relations. By the time Black was ready to ascend to the position of administrator, she was well prepared to be the COO of the entire organization. Clay makes it a point to divide her time equally between the hospital, the rehabilitation center, and the nursing home to ensure that all aspects of the operation are working cohesively and present the same high-quality presence to its customer community. She is on the board of advisors to the local nursing school and is an instructor in the organization's GED program.

Joe Tunney, previously the assistant administrator of human resources for MCH, is currently the chief administrative officer (CAO) of the entire corporation. In addition to human resources and personnel administration, he administers certain operational aspects of the hospital, specifically security and cafeteria operations. The reason for this is that both the security force and cafeteria workers are the only unionized components left within the Maryville organization, and Tunney's career path prior to Maryville was at a major food-service organization. Tunney has a training and development specialist, a wage and compensation administrator, and two employee relations specialists working for him and, like Tyson and Clay, he ensures that he spends equal time at each of the three facilities. He has a bachelor's degree in industrial psychology and a master's in business administration, and is very active in the Historical Society of Douglas County and as a director of the Oak City Oaks, a minor-league baseball team and popular source of entertainment in the summer months. In addition to managing the hospital's extensive on-site education program, Tunney serves as an instructor in the entry-level business courses sponsored by Douglas Community College, both at the facility and on campus. His on-campus activities provide the side benefit of being able to recruit hourly and semiskilled personnel from the local community who are potentially solid Maryville employees.

Fontana makes it a point to meet with his management council every two weeks and schedules meetings at other times only when dictated by pressing circumstances. Although adamant about not letting his managers suffer from "meeting burnout," he does, however, spend at least a half-hour every week meeting formally or informally with each one of his direct reports. Additionally, Fontana makes it a point never to have a cup of coffee in his office. Rather, he has coffee in the cafeteria with an employee or with a department head in the department head's office. Fontana uses this "management-by-coffee" process to talk with as many members of the organization as possible. He normally spends three days at the hospital and one day each at the retirement facility and the rehabilitation facility.

Managers and Supervisors

The remainder of Maryville's management staff and supervisory personnel are well tenured and form a chain of command averaging five to seven direct reports from entry-level hourly workers up to the management council. A recent wage survey of the Pacific Northwest indicates that all salaries at Maryville are in the top-25 percentile in all areas. Turnover is approximately 10 percent and, as in many other institutions, recruitment and retention are most difficult in the areas of physical therapy, pharmacy, nursing, and certain skilled hourly positions.

☐ Progressive Management Strategies at Maryville

The Maryville mission and values statements embrace many important standards of ethical commitment, corporate culture, and approaches to management in serving the Maryville customer/patient or customer/ resident. The statements read as follows:

Mission: To provide top-quality health care services to all members of our community who are in need of our services.

Values:

1. Our customer/patient is at the top of our organizational chart.
2. Every employee is a valued asset and is equal in importance.
3. We are in the people business; the human touch is our best product.
4. Nobody succeeds in our organization unless we all succeed.
5. The dignity of all patients and employees will never be compromised.
6. We are a community public trust.
7. Quality is more than a cliché.
8. Compassion is a job requirement.
9. Learning and growing are job benefits.
10. Excellence of job execution is an everyday objective.

To enforce these standards daily, the organization employs a complete set of progressive management strategies, starting with tactics directed toward the two most important people in the Maryville scheme of operations—the customer and the individual employee. In the estimation of the board and the CEO, Maryville historically has been successful due to the uncommon bond between the Douglas County residents and the Maryville employees. Therefore, it is essential that a starting point in its progressive management strategy is the publication and publicity of the management mission statement and values, or credo, to increase awareness of the mission and values among both customers and employees.

Under the direction of Helen Clay, many marketing efforts have been made to publicize the Maryville mission. These include methods commonly used by many health care organizations, such as displaying the credo in the reception area and throughout the facilities of all Maryville components. Perhaps more creatively, Clay has employed other programs to present the Maryville mission to its customer community. These include a health fair program, which is presented at all the local grammar schools, high schools, and other meeting places throughout the Douglas County area. The program includes the participation of several staff nurses and other Maryville professionals in conducting blood tests and other routine procedures and presenting a well-conceived program of health information on current trends, fitness, stress management, and other pertinent issues. Program participants receive a manual, which contains the Maryville credo and mission statement as well as a list of services provided by the Maryville organization.

Another effort includes having Maryville emergency personnel and related medical professionals posted at various sporting events throughout the customer community. Their presence, which does not jeopardize hospital emergency operations, has been managed with Tyson's assistance and his contacts in the local sports community.

In a similar fashion, the Maryville organization has sponsored "Health Day" for the Oak City Oaks, which included giveaways of inexpensive painters' hats and other promotional items at the gates to all baseball fans who live in the Douglas County community. This again provides a strong presence within the community and reinforces the organization's perception of being a vital part of the community.

Of special interest to Clay is Maryville's participation with the local nursing school, located in Brownsville. This nursing school is Clay's alma mater, and she has maintained ties through her teaching activities and has placed an inordinate number of nurses at the facility following their graduation. By employing these graduates at the Maryville organization, she not only has developed a resource for recruitment but has maintained a sense that the nursing staff at Maryville is the "community's own."

With Fontana and the board's approval, Clay has recently extended fiscal and equipment resources to the nursing school, such as scholarships, internships, and operational equipment. The operational equipment breeds a degree of familiarity with the nursing students, a familiarity that can naturally be continued if they embark on their careers at Maryville. The scholarships and internships likewise encourage a familiarity with the organization, the facilities, and "the Maryville way of nursing."

Several years ago, in the interest of maximizing community awareness of the facility, Fontana constructed a citizen advisory panel composed of citizens from the community who would act in an advisory role to the hospital's activities and overall direction. The panel provided several useful suggestions, which included a new parking scheme for the hospital and an open house for the customer community.

Whereas most open houses connote a recruitment device to the health care executive, these open houses had a dual purpose. Their primary purpose was to provide a quarterly exhibition of all the hospital's activities and a presentation of the aforementioned on-site health fair program. The secondary purpose was to provide an opportunity for prospective employees to see the facility, talk to various representatives of the organization, and present an application or resumé for employment consideration. The open house meant the participation of most of MCH's employees, but the Saturday overtime pay to various nonexempt individuals was easily offset by the reduction in recruitment costs and the increased interest from the customer community.

Another suggestion from the citizen advisory panel, which was confirmed by other members of the public responding to marketing surveys generated by Helen Clay's office, was the establishment of an "Ethics in Action" program. This program consisted of several discussion sessions held throughout the organization in which individual employees had an opportunity to discuss ethics and MCH's values. In each case, meeting participants were encouraged to suggest how MCH's organizational ethics could be better represented and put into action. An outcome of these sessions included the installation of an employee referral recruitment program, similar to that discussed in chapter 7. Appendix D contains more information about the construction of such a program.

The citizen advisory panel also had the opportunity to participate in the bimonthly management council meetings, which were also attended by members of the board of directors. Fontana used this time to have his managers present a "show-and-tell" presentation about each of their respective five areas of Maryville's overall management. The managers had the option of presenting the material themselves, exhibiting a new project or procedure, or delegating the presentation to one of their respective reporting managers or supervisors. This allowed the development of the presentational skills of all of these managers, as well as providing straightforward communication to all members of the Maryville community. It also provided Fontana and the board of directors an opportunity to discuss specific issues with the citizen advisory panel and elicit their suggestions and input on the most advantageous way of pursuing the specific business objectives.

In respect to increasing employee commitment to the mission and credo of Maryville Community Healthcare, Fontana started with a novel idea. He took the main objectives of the Maryville credo and had them reduced to the size of a one-inch-square miniplaque. These miniplaques were then laminated with a special durable substance by a specialty firm owned by a member of the board of directors, made into key chains, and given to the employees.

To take the idea one step further, Fontana implemented a monthly employee newsletter, which would be circulated throughout the entire organization. Each issue reported general news about the organization and included a letter from Fontana as an editorial piece. No less than 75 percent of each issue was generated by individual employees from all three facilities. Articles spotlighted new programs, high levels of performance achievement, graduates of the Maryville on-site education program, promotions and transfers, and other important employee achievements. The newsletter also included news about the community that was pertinent to the hospital and invariably contained coupons or special offers through the employee purchase program. It also provided a forum for questions from employees and, in some cases, customer/patients or residents, to be answered by respective members of the organization.

A special feature of the newsletter was the "suggestion of the month" program. Inaugurated by Cynthia Rose, this program gave every member of the Maryville community—employee or customer—the opportunity to receive a $500 savings bond for the best suggestion received by Fontana's office within a given month. Some award-winning suggestions included the following:

- A "night meals program," where a local food distributor contributed overstocked items to the hospital cafeteria at the close of the night shift at midnight. This food was then used by the hospital cafeteria to provide nutritious meals free of cost to employees working the "graveyard shift" from midnight to 8 a.m. The program helped these employees avoid foods of dubious nutritional content while providing the food-service company an opportunity to contribute to community needs and benefit from positive publicity.
- A day-care center, which was suggested by a resident at the Maryville Retirement Center. A major problem at the main hospital had been child care for single parents or parents of dual-income families. Many of the residents at the Maryville Retirement Community were vibrant and eager to work and participate in something meaningful; therefore, a day-care center was established at the retirement center, the rehabilitation center, and the hospital, all of which were staffed by qualified residents at the retirement center. These residents were compensated by a proportional decrease on their monthly bill, and because many were parents or grandparents, they had experience in providing high-quality child care.
- The establishment of a cafeteria line adjusted to wheelchair height, allowing individuals, notably at the rehabilitation facility, to have meals with a visitor or loved one rather than within the confines of their room or in other specially designated areas. This suggestion was provided by a dietary employee.
- Training in common Spanish phrases. This program was suggested jointly by a customer/patient and an employee, who ultimately both received savings bonds as rewards for their suggestions. Because the Mega-Tech organization, as well as Linial Aircraft, employed many individuals for whom English was a second language, quite often Maryville personnel needed to be able to speak in Spanish. To meet this need, a Spanish-speaking employee devised a list of 25 conversational exchanges—for example, a visitor looking for a patient's room. Each employee who mastered these phrases was awarded a certain amount of points on his or her performance evaluation. This also made the hospital more user friendly to these individuals and demonstrated commitment to all customer/patients.

Other steps taken by Fontana as a result of the employee/patient suggestion program included a CEO hot-line number, a phone line installed to an answering machine in Fontana's office. Published in the employee newsletter every month, this number was accessible to all employees at all times so they could share information or suggestions with Fontana in a confidential manner. While having to maintain a sense of balance in reviewing some of the comments provided, Fontana did discover an employee perception of "elitism" due to the numbered parking spot system employed by the hospital for years. The system was soon eliminated, particularly after several employees called with the same complaint.

The hot line also revealed an increased demand for more hospital-sponsored employee outings, particularly tickets to the Oak City Oaks baseball games and other local events. These suggestions were followed up by Fontana himself, as he was able to provide a bartering system of exchanging advertising space in the employee newsletter for tickets, which were then distributed by individual managers to employees who provided stellar performance.

Central to Maryville's successful employee relations programs is the high quality of the management manual used by each supervisor, department head, and executive within the organization. Devised by James Black, Joe Tunney, and a representative committee of employees from throughout the Maryville organization, the manual contains guidelines and instructions on how to administer Maryville's management programs, specifically its employee performance evaluation and compensation programs.

Several years ago, Maryville implemented the use of an incentive-based compensation program for all employees under which each employee was given the opportunity to set goals jointly with his or her supervisor for overall annual performance. The employee would submit a set of 10 goals, based on the characteristics of his or her job description, for ratification by the supervisor and inclusion in a performance planning document. Also included in the document was a set of organizational mission objectives and work personality characteristics, or values, which are also graded and factored into the overall performance rating. The opportunity for the employee to participate in the performance evaluation process, as well as to contribute expertise and insight into particular work areas, is considered a major reason for the low (10 percent) annual turnover figure throughout the organization.

The performance evaluation process at Maryville also includes a personnel development program for all employees and managers. As explained in chapters 7 and 8, the employee or manager's performance, potential, and promotability is discussed and analyzed by the supervisor during each rating period. The employee or manager is given a forthright estimation of his or her potential within the organization and provided with a personnel development plan for training and development within the given job.

Personnel and management development at Maryville not only enhances the knowledge and skills of all staff members but helps to ensure that the organization's bonus dollars are distributed throughout the organization. Each employee, from the lowest tiers of the hourly ranks to the CEO's office, is eligible for bonus payments at the end of the year based on individual performance and the organization's overall achievements.

Perhaps unique to the Maryville approach to management, and listed among the motivators in appendix C, is a system for awarding bonuses to employees with long tenures at the organization. In combination with Maryville's other pay-for-performance approaches to compensation, longevity bonuses encourage the maximum utilization of employee talents and encourage optimum performance from every member. The collective effect is that Maryville is perceived throughout its community as being a progressive employer that rewards outstanding performance.

Other programs utilized by Maryville to reflect its progressive attitude toward management include:

- An employee cafeteria in which meals are discounted and in some cases free (such as for overtime workers).
- A new parking area close to the rear of the hospital and immediately adjacent to an employee entrance. This eliminated the perception of elitism and made getting to work more convenient for all employees. Each of the three Maryville sites has such a parking scheme.
- An employee purchase program, open to all employees. A wide range of catalog items is available at discounted rates.
- An employee assistance program, which provides counseling to employees or their family members. By utilizing the clinical psychologist on staff at Maryville, the organization provides a low-overhead vital service.
- Outplacement for an employee who leaves voluntarily or as a result of a termination.
- A complete education program throughout the Maryville system, augmented by an employee development program that includes training courses in a variety of technical, management, and business subject areas. Courses range from communication skills to time management, stress management, and management techniques, all presented by various members of Joe Tunney's staff, and available to all members of the organization. Each training program has as part of its educational theme various aspects of the Maryville credo. Thus, a synergistic effect of two elements of the credo—mission and education—are addressed pointedly by one major program. Tunney's staff conducts several surveys

throughout the year to determine what type of training is needed, and whether individual or group strategies are needed to meet suggested training needs and desires.

☐ Practical Applications

To date, Maryville Community Healthcare Corporation has operated as a successful, independent entity in a very competitive marketplace. Its success and vibrancy, unique among health care institutions, are founded on a very simple principle: In its credo, Maryville describes itself as being a public trust—similar to a fire department, a police department, or an educational system—and as such, charges its employees with a very precious and critical responsibility to its customer community. By implementing a value-driven management system composed of commonsense strategies and intelligent tactics, organizations such as Maryville are destined to set the pace for the progressive delivery of health care in the turbulent 1990s.

The following practical applications are offered to help you integrate the lessons of the case study into your own management setting:

1. Use the case study as a teaching/training tool in staff development efforts and team discussions.
2. Determine what segments of the case study can be directly applied to your organization or department.
3. Use the case study as a discussion topic in board meetings or executive retreats.
4. Compare Maryville's mission and value statements to your organization's.
5. What would you do differently if you were any member of the Maryville organization?
6. Some health care managers believe that this case study is a model for any community hospital. What three major ideas does it contribute to your frame of reference?
7. Garner your employees' perceptions and ideas about the case study for potential suggestions.
8. Predict the future for Maryville. What challenges do you believe it will face in the near future?
9. What steps would you take as a Maryville competitor?
10. In general, how does Maryville compare with your organization? What makes "the difference" that enables it to be successful?

Appendixes

☐ Appendix A

Organizational Peformance Values

This appendix contains the 20 performance values discussed in chapter 3. Each performance value is defined and presented in terms of criterion-based assessment factors, that is, positive practical actions and negative counteractions.

Furthermore, each value is augmented by a list of questions or "cues," which can be used in interviewing and selecting new employees or in conducting organizational audits of existing and current staff. Pertinent interviewee or employee responses to questions can be recorded in the spaces labeled "clues."

The organizational audit can be completed by filling out the progressive management factors work sheet that follows each list of questions. Space is provided in sections I and III of the form for listing positive and negative role models from within the organization. The space in section II is provided for listing the benefits brought to the organization by the positive role models. The space in section IV is provided for listing the risks to the organization generated by the negative role models. Notes for taking corrective action among specific individuals can be recorded in section V. A sample work sheet that has been filled out by the author can be found in figure A-1.

At the end of each of the four sets of values (personal values, humanistic standards, business norms, and executive principles) is a personal review and action chart for self- examination, reflection, and further action planning.

Figure A-1.   Sample Progressive Management Factors Work Sheet

Knowledge: Constantly pursues growth and development activities that strengthen business knowledge, technical acumen, and personal enhancement; realizes that there is something to be learned every day and in every situation, and that attainment of as much knowledge as possible is a responsibility and requirement of ethical leadership.

   I. Positive Organizational Role Models:
      1. E. Ross, Nursing
      2. G. Calvin, Pharmacy
      3. D. L. Miller, Radiology

  II. Organization-Specific Positive Benefits:
      a. Breadth of knowledge across organization, as well as basic competency
      b. Depth of knowledge in all technical areas
      c. Increasing effectiveness and efficiency of work

 III. Negative Organizational Role Models:
      1. G. Zimmerman, Public Relations
      2. K. DeLuca, Assistant Administrator
      3. J. Kimble, Planning

 IV. Organization-Specific Negative Risks:
      a. Incompetence at key levels and in key areas of expertise
      b. Politics instead of performance
      c. Poor developmental role models

  V. Action Notes:
     III/1,2,3: Address through performance evaluation and corrective education
     III/2:   Potential probation. Previous counseling has not produced results

☐ Personal Values: Ethical Standards Instilled in Individuals through Their Upbringing, Education, and Experience

Decency: Consistently demonstrates a basic sense of propriety as it applies to the human factor in the workplace; never places the desire to "do the right thing" in a secondary role in the workplace.

Fortitude: Brings a sound, unpretentious quality of courage to the everyday workplace that enables the capacity to make tough decisions and seek the most ethical solution to any business challenge; is patient in obtaining solid results and steadfast in constructing ethically optimum plans.

Industry: Understands the need to dedicate one's efforts to maximum effectiveness and efficiency every day and in all business circumstances; readily accepts the daily responsibility of being a role model of quality output and optimum effort and production.

Integrity: Incorporates honor, truthfulness, and sincerity into an everyday work philosophy; is uncompromising in seeking the factual evidence in every situation and resolute in providing upright stances and credible data in all situations.

Knowledge: Constantly pursues growth and development activities that strengthen business knowledge, technical acumen, and personal enhancement; realizes that there is something to be learned every day and in every situation, and that attainment of as much knowledge as possible is a responsibility and requirement of ethical leadership.

☐ Personal Values

Decency

Consistently demonstrates a basic sense of propriety as it applies to the human factor in the workplace; never places the desire to "do the right thing" in a secondary role in the workplace.

Positive Practical Actions:

- Uses personal action as a daily reminder of the value of basic decency in the workplace
- Treats all personnel—from housekeepers to the CEO—as valued, important human beings and organizational players
- Uses appropriate language and tact when describing people, no matter who they are or what they have done
- Never lets the quest for decency become a hindrance in dealing with distasteful individuals
- Has a practical sense of right and wrong as it applies to the health care workplace
- Does not let actions away from the job reflect poorly on the organization
- Never allows sense of decency to become sanctimonious or questioned as hypocritical due to actions

Negative Counteractions:

- Demonstrates a sense of decency only if it is convenient to the business situation at hand
- Lacks practical knowledge of what is good or bad in a health care business situation
- Regards hourly employees as stupid or has trouble relating to ethnics or minorities
- Is decent only when dealing with someone he or she likes personally
- Demonstrates a sense of decency only when something can be gained from the situation
- Is perceived throughout the organization as a phony

☐ Cue Sheet: Personal Values

Decency

Cue #1: Often, the terms *decency* or *doing the right thing* are used as clichés. Tell me about a situation you had to manage where those terms took on meaningful importance.

Clues: a. _____

b. _____

Cue #2: How does the quality of decency fit into your managerial philosophy?

Clues: a. _____

b. _____

Cue #3: Explain the importance of basic decency in the health care workplace.

Clues: a. _____

b. _____

Cue #4: Why are hourly employees so integral to the success of a health care organization?

Clues: a. _____

b. _____

Cue #5: Describe an employee who exhibited an innate sense of "doing the right thing" in every work situation.

Clues: a. _____

b. _____

☐ Progressive Management Factors Work Sheet: Personal Values

Decency: Consistently demonstrates a basic sense of propriety as it applies to the human factor in the workplace; never places the desire to "do the right thing" in a secondary role in the workplace.

I. Positive Organizational Role Models:

    1. _____

    2. _____

    3. _____

II. Organization-Specific Positive Benefits:

    a. _____

    b. _____

    c. _____

III. Negative Organizational Role Models:

    1. _____

    2. _____

    3. _____

IV. Organization-Specific Negative Risks:

    a. _____

    b. _____

    c. _____

V. Action Notes:

☐ Personal Values

Fortitude

Brings a sound, unpretentious quality of courage to the everyday workplace that enables the capacity to make tough decisions and seek the most ethical solution to any business challenge; is patient in obtaining solid results and steadfast in constructing ethically optimum plans.

Positive Practical Actions:

- Never shies away from making the "tough call"
- Examines every conceivable angle of an issue before making a decision that might adversely affect the work life of an employee
- Has true courage of convictions, as evidenced by everyday work actions
- Has a history of work experience and general background that indicate a propensity for making correct decisions without regard for popularity
- Is not easily swayed by strong counterpersonalities or dubious adverse arguments
- Takes as much time as appropriate to examine the rationale for decisions or position on certain issues
- Demands high ethical standards of conduct from employees, no matter what their technical talent or job market value might be

Negative Counteractions:

- Makes strong ethical statements in high-profile situations, but not "backstage"
- Has strength of character that is suspect in eyes of employees and coworkers
- Will make an initial "tough call" but not support it with substantial action
- Is impatient in examining situations and critical information; takes the quickest, most expedient route without consideration of long-term effects
- Makes ethically strong statements but does not take ethically strong action
- Has a work/academic background that is replete with examples of ethically questionable actions
- Supports others in the organization who are not of the strongest ethical fiber

☐ Cue Sheet: Personal Values

Fortitude

Cue #1: What was the toughest ethically based decision you had to make in a health care management situation?

Clues: a. _____

b. _____

Cue #2: Define *fortitude* for me, as it relates to your everyday responsibilities.

Clues: a. _____

b. _____

Cue #3: Describe a situation in which you had to encourage someone to make a "tough call."

Clues: a. _____

b. _____

Cue #4: What methods have you utilized to instill a sense of fortitude in your reporting staff?

Clues: a. _____

b. _____

Cue #5: Why should fortitude be part of a health care manager's daily strategy?

Clues: a. _____

b. _____

☐ Progressive Management Factors Work Sheet: Personal Values

Fortitude: Brings a sound, unpretentious quality of courage to the everyday workplace that enables the capacity to make tough decisions and seek the most ethical solution to any business challenge; is patient in obtaining solid results and steadfast in constructing ethically optimum plans.

I. Positive Organizational Role Models:

1. _____

2. _____

3. _____

II. Organization-Specific Positive Benefits:

a. _____

b. _____

c. _____

III. Negative Organizational Role Models:

1. _____

2. _____

3. _____

IV. Organization-Specific Negative Risks:

a. _____

b. _____

c. _____

V. Action Notes:

☐ Personal Values

Industry

Understands the need to dedicate one's efforts to maximum effectiveness and efficiency every day and in all business circumstances; readily accepts the daily responsibility of being a role model of quality output and optimum effort and production.

Positive Practical Actions:

- Has a work ethic that serves as an example for all members of the organization
- Works at a top level on all projects, not just those of particular interest
- Makes the most of all opportunities, from weekly meetings and routine "administrivia" to emergency situations and high-visibility opportunities for action
- Never accepts anything but the best possible effort from subordinates
- Challenges self to always seek the "higher ground" with respect to effort and results
- Understands that "half-stepping" on the part of the individual or anyone in his or her chain of command cheats the organization and the customer/patient
- Realizes that the health care business forum is no place for laziness, apathy, or politicking as opposed to results

Negative Counteractions:

- Exhibits selective industriousness; works hard at things that have high visibility or are of major interest but slacks off on other activities
- Puts a premium on politics and power as opposed to production
- Does not project a creditable presence of industry and dedication to excellence
- Communicates, through action and example, that "coasting" is acceptable behavior
- Does not realize that laziness and apathy can be a contributing factor toward inadequate health care service
- Coddles employees who are not highly motivated toward maximum productivity
- Has a work ethic that is unsuitable for the demands of health care

☐ Cue Sheet: Personal Values

Industry

Cue #1: Describe a particularly industrious manager you've worked with or worked for.

Clues: a. _____

b. _____

Cue #2: Describe a particularly industrious person who worked for you at some point in your career.

Clues: a. _____

b. _____

Cue #3: Describe a work situation you had to remedy where lack of industry had taken hold.

Clues: a. _____

b. _____

Cue #4: How do you approach meetings and paperwork, which seem to inundate every health care manager/executive?

Clues: a. _____

b. _____

Cue #5: Describe a work group/organization you're familiar with that truly engenders a sense of industry.

Clues: a. _____

b. _____

☐ Progressive Management Factors Work Sheet: Personal Values

Industry: Understands the need to dedicate one's efforts to maximum effectiveness and efficiency every day and in all business circumstances; readily accepts the daily responsibility of being a role model of quality output and optimum effort and production.

I. Positive Organizational Role Models:

   1. _____

   2. _____

   3. _____

II. Organization-Specific Positive Benefits:

   a. _____

   b. _____

   c. _____

III. Negative Organizational Role Models:

   1. _____

   2. _____

   3. _____

IV. Organization-Specific Negative Risks:

   a. _____

   b. _____

   c. _____

V. Action Notes:

☐ Personal Values

Integrity

Incorporates honor, truthfulness, and sincerity into an everyday work philosophy; is uncompromising in seeking the factual evidence in every situation and resolute in providing upright stances and data in all situations.

Positive Practical Actions:

- Presents facts and credible figures as part of rationale for decision making
- Refuses to accept opinions or viewpoints blindly without substantiation
- Demands that subordinates make decisions based on fact and evidence, not conjecture or opinion
- Seeks solutions independently when appropriate; does not rely on popular support to take a stand
- Is honorable in all business dealings
- Is unafraid of relaying "bad news" directly but compassionately
- Maintains a record of unquestionable honesty and communicative candor in key business dealings
- Tells the whole story, not just the accepted or popular segments

Negative Counteractions:

- Is perceived widely as a "storyteller"
- Lets subordinates "present the 'truth'" to him or her in a creative manner
- Prefaces statements with: "_____ says that . . .," "I think that . . .," "I have a sense that. . . ."
- Uses no factual rationale for actions taken or approaches adopted
- Rarely cites facts, figures, precedence, or situational factors
- Is more interested in acceptance than results, and predicates business philosophy accordingly

☐ Cue Sheet: Personal Values

Integrity

Cue #1:   Often, *integrity* is used as a cliche in management discussions. What realistic meaning does it hold for you?

Clues: a. _____

          b. _____

Cue #2:   Discuss an employee you had to deal with who lacked integrity.

Clues: a. _____

          b. _____

Cue #3:   How do you handle giving someone "bad news"? [The interviewer should try to elicit an example.]

Clues: a. _____

          b. _____

Cue #4:   Explain the importance of fundamental integrity in the health care workplace.

Clues: a. _____

          b. _____

Cue #5:   Relate an example of a major turnaround situation you had to manage. How did you know the turnaround was successful?

Clues: a. _____

          b. _____

☐ Progressive Management Factors Work Sheet: Personal Values

Integrity: Incorporates honor, truthfulness, and sincerity into an everyday work philosophy; is uncompromising in seeking the factual evidence in every situation and resolute in providing upright stances and credible data in all situations.

I. Positive Organizational Role Models:

    1. _____

    2. _____

    3. _____

II. Organization-Specific Positive Benefits:

    a. _____

    b. _____

    c. _____

III. Negative Organizational Role Models:

    1. _____

    2. _____

    3. _____

IV. Organization-Specific Negative Risks:

    a. _____

    b. _____

    c. _____

V. Action Notes:

☐ Personal Values

Knowledge

Constantly pursues growth and development activities that strengthen business knowledge, technical acumen, and personal enhancement; realizes that there is something to be learned every day and in every situation and that attainment of as much knowledge as possible is a responsibility and requirement of ethical leadership.

Positive Practical Actions:

- Takes advantage of as many developmental activities as possible, from seminars to enlightening discussions
- Reads as much as possible on significant issues
- Recognizes the learning value in talking to an hourly employee or a customer/patient
- Asks the right questions in all business situations
- Seeks opportunities to understand rationales and philosophies as well as objective facts
- Attempts to gain knowledge in a wide breadth of areas pertinent to managerial responsibility
- Constantly develops a creditable depth of knowledge in key areas of technical responsibility
- Learns from situations, people, and circumstances as much as from books and seminars

Negative Counteractions:

- Thinks he or she "knows it all"
- Is spiteful of the opinions and viewpoints of others
- Never digs beneath the surface of a situation
- Does not take advantage of traditional educational opportunities, for example, seminars, books, conferences, and so forth
- Does not take advantage of nontraditional education, for example, talks with employees, personal involvement, and so forth
- Thinks most people are stupid and intellectually inferior

☐ Cue Sheet: Personal Values

Knowledge

Cue #1: How do you increase your ongoing knowledge of _____
[Choose an aspect or aspects of the interviewee's expertise.]

Clues: a. _____

b. _____

Cue #2: What methods have you utilized to increase your subordinates' professional knowledge?

Clues: a. _____

b. _____

Cue #3: Relate a situation that you learned a great deal from.

Clues: a. _____

b. _____

Cue #4: Give an example of a management situation where your health care/managerial/technical knowledge was a great asset.

Clues: a. _____

b. _____

Cue #5: What's the most important thing you've learned in the past five years?

Clues a. _____

b. _____

☐ Progressive Management Factors Work Sheet: Personal Values

Knowledge: Constantly pursues growth and development activities that strengthen business knowledge, technical acumen, and personal enhancement; realizes that there is something to be learned every day and in every situation and that attainment of as much knowledge as possible is a responsibility and requirement of ethical leadership.

I. Positive Organizational Role Models:

    1. _____

    2. _____

    3. _____

II. Organization-Specific Positive Benefits:

    a. _____

    b. _____

    c. _____

III. Negative Organizational Role Models:

    1. _____

    2. _____

    3. _____

IV. Organization-Specific Negative Risks:

    a. _____

    b. _____

    c. _____

V. Action Notes:

☐ Personal Review and Action Chart: Personal Values

1. Rank your own strength in the personal values, on a scale from 1 to 5 (5: very strong, 4: fairly high, 3: adequate, 2: need some improvement, 1: critical).

   Decency: _____   Integrity: _____

   Fortitude: _____   Knowledge: _____

   Industry: _____

2. Rank the personal values in relative importance to your job (5: vitally important, 4: very important, 3: needed, 2: optional, 1: meaningless).

   Decency: _____   Integrity: _____

   Fortitude: _____   Knowledge: _____

   Industry: _____

3. Rank your organization's effectiveness in the personal values. (Use the same scale as for question #1.)

   Decency: _____   Integrity: _____

   Fortitude: _____   Knowledge: _____

   Industry: _____

4. Rate your boss relative to the personal values. (Use the same scale as for question #1.)

   Decency: _____   Integrity: _____

   Fortitude: _____   Knowledge: _____

   Industry: _____

5. List specific positive and practical actions you will now undertake:

   a. _____

   b. _____

6. List specific negative counteractions you will try to eliminate:

   a. _____

   b. _____

☐ Humanistic Standards: Value-Based Guidelines for Understanding, Accepting, and Relating to Other People

Allegiance: Demonstrates through words and actions a fidelity to helping those in need and supporting others engaged in the provision of superior health care; is unwavering in assisting those in need and giving maximum effort in both individual and group activities that benefit the organization.

Compassion: Sensitivity toward others is reflected in acceptance of varied personalities, appreciation of cultural differences, and a genuine affection for people that transcends clichés and superficial statements and is expressed in continuous action both on and off the job.

Dignity: Provides all employees the opportunity to grow and develop full professional potential; respects every employee and promotes a workplace climate where each professional is treated as the most important asset.

Introspection: Constantly challenges self to attain the highest degree of professional achievement and maintain the best ethical standards in all situations; is consistent in thinking through important issues, balancing consequences with action, and tempering firmness with humanistic consideration.

Spirit: Manifests a self-generated positive attitude toward the health care industry, a vitality toward everyday responsibilities, and an incessant desire to become a better professional and person; has an infectious enthusiasm for the health care workplace and its important mission.

□ Humanistic Standards

Allegiance

Demonstrates through words and actions a fidelity to helping those in need and supporting others engaged in the provision of superior health care; is unwavering in assisting those in need and giving maximum effort in both individual and group activities that benefit the organization.

Positive Practical Actions:

- Is eminently capable of being trusted to help and support those in need
- Displays a notable degree of loyalty to those who are deserving
- Looks for opportunities to help others who can benefit from assistance, support, and guidance
- Willingly acts as a mentor to inexperienced personnel
- Helps those who help themselves; does not "carry" reluctant, uninspired, or marginal players
- Has a steadfast dedication to encouraging reporting personnel toward peak performance and optimum professional contribution
- Is capable of trusting deserving others and rendering trust and confidence when appropriate

Negative Counteractions:

- Is suspicious of most people, to the point of being paranoid
- Expects the worst from people in general
- Sincerely believes that most fellow professionals are incompetent or not as dedicated as he or she is
- Sees others' allegiance as a sign of weakness and seeks to exploit it
- Helps only those who can directly and quickly "pay back the favor"
- Often speaks in negative terms about others and is quick to cite the weaknesses of coworkers, subordinates, or superiors
- Cannot be trusted to "do the right thing" in most situations; has work actions and philosophies that breed suspicion in others

☐ Cue Sheet: Humanistic Standards

Allegiance

Cue #1: Give an example of your participation as a mentor to some-
         one in your current/last organization.

Clues: a. _____

         b. _____

Cue #2: Tell about a work group you had to manage that lacked a true
         sense of allegiance.

Clues: a. _____

         b. _____

Cue #3: Define *allegiance* as it relates to the health care workplace.

Clues: a. _____

         b. _____

Cue #4: Do you sometimes find it difficult to trust others in a work
         situation?

Clues: a. _____

         b. _____

Cue #5: What methods have you utilized to inspire allegiance among
         your reporting staff?

Clues: a. _____

         b. _____

☐ Progressive Management Factors Work Sheet: Humanistic Standards

Allegiance: Demonstrates through words and actions a fidelity to helping those in need and supporting others engaged in the provision of superior health care; is unwavering in assisting those in need and giving maximum effort in both individual and group activities that benefit the organization.

I. Positive Organizational Role Models:

    1. _____

    2. _____

    3. _____

II. Organization-Specific Positive Benefits:

    a. _____

    b. _____

    c. _____

III. Negative Organizational Role Models:

    1. _____

    2. _____

    3. _____

IV. Organization-Specific Negative Risks:

    a. _____

    b. _____

    c. _____

V. Action Notes:

☐ Humanistic Standards

Compassion

Sensitivity toward others is reflected in acceptance of varied personalities, appreciation of cultural differences, and a genuine affection for people that transcends clichés and superficial statements and is expressed in continuous action on and off the job.

Positive Practical Actions:

- Listens closely and weighs decisions carefully when confronted with a people-intensive situation
- Demands workplace fairness for all personnel and exercises appropriate judgment in enforcing related standards
- Has a fundamental respect for all people, and does not differentiate on educational level, race, culture, or other personal issues in pursuing fair action
- Does not sermonize on sensitive issues, but lets actions and personal style set the standard and tell the story
- Understands that all people are different and deserve individual consideration in applying universal fairness
- Does not coddle or "carry" one employee to the point of alienating truly committed players
- Can converse easily with anyone and understand a variety of perceptions and viewpoints expressed by others

Negative Counteractions:

- Talks a good game but does not prove sensitivity through actions
- Gravitates toward meaningless clichés and negative stereotypes when discussing others
- Rarely makes the time to discuss problems with those who need help
- Only has time for people he or she likes or can relate to due to similar backgrounds/philosophies
- Provides opportunities only for those of similar backgrounds/philosophies
- Perceived as not being people-oriented, someone interested only in the "bottom line"

☐ Cue Sheet: Humanistic Standards

Compassion

Cue #1: *Compassion* is a word that has many meanings in health care parlance. What does it mean to you?

Clues: a. _____

b. _____

Cue #2: Have you worked in organizations characterized by cultural diversity?

Clues: a. _____

b. _____

Cue #3: Who is the most compassionate member of your current staff?

Clues: a. _____

b. _____

Cue #4: Define compassion, as it relates to everyday health care work activities.

Clues: a. _____

b. _____

Cue #5: Tell about a situation you had to manage that required inordinate compassion.

Clues: a. _____

b. _____

☐ Progressive Management Factors Work Sheet: Humanistic Standards

Compassion: Sensitivity toward others is reflected in acceptance of varied personalities, appreciation of cultural differences, and a genuine affection for people that transcends clichés and superficial statements and is expressed in continuous action both on and off the job.

I. Positive Organizational Role Models:

   1. _____

   2. _____

   3. _____

II. Organization-Specific Positive Benefits:

   a. _____

   b. _____

   c. _____

III. Negative Organizational Role Models:

   1. _____

   2. _____

   3. _____

IV. Organization-Specific Negative Risks:

   a. _____

   b. _____

   c. _____

V. Action Notes:

☐ Humanistic Standards

Dignity

Provides all employees the opportunity to grow and develop full professional potential; respects every employee and promotes a workplace climate where each professional is treated as the most important asset.

Positive Practical Actions

- Respects all members of the organization, from housekeepers to board members
- Renders respect in the same manner in which it is given
- Makes decisions expediently and in a manner that will maintain the employee's dignity
- Charges managers with the responsibility of ensuring individual employee dignity
- Seeks out opportunities to develop employees as much as possible on both a professional and interpersonal level
- Solicits information from a variety of sources on maintaining and increasing the dignity quotient throughout the organization
- Understands and reinforces through action the importance of individual dignity to the overall success and cohesiveness of the health care organization

Negative Counteractions:

- Is unfairly selective in giving respect to individuals
- Lets individual dignity steadily take a backseat to profits
- Allows policies and actions that rarely take into account the interests and development of the individual
- Allows policies based on politics, which in turn do not take into account the issue of personal dignity
- Ignores input on dignity issues; does not take such data into consideration when making decisions
- Actions do not reflect respect toward others' viewpoints and beliefs

☐ Cue Sheet: Humanistic Standards

Dignity

Cue #1:   How do you ensure that dignity is a meaningful part of every-
          day work activities?

Clues: a. _____

          b. _____

Cue #2:   Have you ever had to remedy a situation where an individual
          failed to respect the dignity of another employee?

Clues: a. _____

          b. _____

Cue #3:   How important are politics in a health care organization?

Clues: a. _____

          b. _____

Cue #4:   *Respect* has become almost a cliché in management texts. How
          does it apply in the management equation?

Clues: a. _____

          b. _____

Cue #5:   What negative consequences have you seen occur in a work-
          place that fails to value the dignity and respect the rights of
          individual employees?

Clues: a. _____

          b. _____

☐ Progressive Management Factors Work Sheet: Humanistic Standards

Dignity: Provides all employees the opportunity to grow and develop full professional potential; respects every employee and promotes a workplace climate where each professional is treated as the most important asset.

I. Positive Organizational Role Models:

    1. _____

    2. _____

    3. _____

II. Organization-Specific Positive Benefits:

    a. _____

    b. _____

    c. _____

III. Negative Organizational Role Models:

    1. _____

    2. _____

    3. _____

IV. Organization-Specific Negative Risks:

    a. _____

    b. _____

    c. _____

V. Action Notes:

☐ Humanistic Standards

Introspection

Constantly challenges self to attain the highest degree of professional achievement and maintain the best ethical standards in all situations; is consistent in thinking through important issues, balancing consequences with action, and tempering firmness with humanistic considerations.

Positive Practical Actions:

- Always gives proper consideration to all significant factors prior to making a decision
- Is his or her "own toughest critic," without becoming negative or risking loss of self-confidence
- Thinks in terms of the means to an end, not just the end result
- Can understand data and decision-making rationale from one point progressively to the next
- Can objectively understand his or her own developmental needs as well as those of others
- Understands the basic motivation, professional needs, and career desires of others
- Has a good depth of thought as well as a breadth of knowledge of coworkers and subordinates

Negative Counteractions:

- Is perceived as being "shallow"; not a deep thinker or a particularly thoughtful leader
- Is self-centered as opposed to self-aware
- Is unaware of how others perceive him or her; does not really care about their perceptions in this regard
- Is more concerned about how others see him or her than on how he or she is perceived
- Never thinks about the long-term effects of a decision, only the short-term, high-profile results
- Is introspective only about issues that affect personal income/professional prestige

☐ Cue Sheet: Humanistic Standards

Introspection

Cue #1: Do you consider yourself to be your own toughest critic?

Clues: a. _____

b. _____

Cue #2: Who was the "deepest thinker" you ever worked with/for or who worked for you?

Clues: a. _____

b. _____

Cue #3: Explain the importance of being introspective as a health care manager.

Clues: a. _____

b. _____

Cue #4: What are some of your developmental needs/opportunities for growth?

Clues: a. _____

b. _____

Cue #5: What motivates you?

Clues: a. _____

b. _____

☐ Progressive Management Factors Work Sheet: Humanistic Standards

Introspection: Constantly challenges self to attain the highest degree of professional achievement and maintain the best ethical standards in all situations; is consistent in thinking through important issues, balancing consequences with action, and tempering firmness with humanistic considerations.

I. Positive Organizational Role Models:

    1. _____

    2. _____

    3. _____

II. Organization-Specific Positive Benefits:

    a. _____

    b. _____

    c. _____

III. Negative Organizational Role Models:

    1. _____

    2. _____

    3. _____

IV. Organization-Specific Negative Risks:

    a. _____

    b. _____

    c. _____

V. Action Notes:

□ Humanistic Standards

Spirit

Manifests a self-generated positive attitude toward the health care industry, a vitality toward everyday responsibilities, and an incessant desire to become a better professional and person; has an infectious enthusiasm for the health care workplace and its important mission.

Positive Practical Actions:

- Maintains a steady, upbeat attitude as appropriately and consistently as possible
- Has a well-founded, agreeable sense of humor
- Acts as a source of positive motivation and encouragement for others
- Takes pride in the accomplishment of staff and is happy for others' success
- Provides a living example of the adage, "quitters never win and winners never quit"
- Acts as though his or her work role is a privilege, not a burden
- Is motivated by things other than money and prestige
- Genuinely displays respect and affection for others

Negative Counteractions:

- Has very "high highs" and very "low lows"
- Has a "bad attitude," which affects individual performance as well as the outlook of others
- Lacks a sense of humor
- Immediately cites the "bad side" of anything
- Is motivated primarily by rewards to self
- Is usually argumentative, negative, contrary, or contrite when confronted by a new or changing situation
- Sees job as an undeserved burden

☐ Cue Sheet: Humanistic Standards

Spirit

Cue #1: How do you engender a sense of spirit in your work group?

Clues: a. _____

          b. _____

Cue #2: Tell about a former boss who was particularly effective in creat-
         ing a strong sense of spirit among his/her charges.

Clues: a. _____

          b. _____

Cue #3: Describe an organization you're familiar with that had a strong,
         cohesive sense of spirit.

Clues: a. _____

          b. _____

Cue #4: How do you motivate your reporting staff?

Clues: a. _____

          b. _____

Cue #5: How do you remain upbeat in your everyday responsibilities?

Clues: a. _____

          b. _____

☐ Progressive Management Factors Work Sheet: Humanistic Standards

Spirit: Manifests a self-generated positive attitude toward the health care industry, a vitality toward everyday responsibilities, and an incessant desire to become a better professional and person; has an infectious enthusiasm for the health care workplace and its important mission.

I. Positive Organizational Role Models:

    1. _____

    2. _____

    3. _____

II. Organization-Specific Positive Benefits:

    a. _____

    b. _____

    c. _____

III. Negative Organizational Role Models:

    1. _____

    2. _____

    3. _____

IV. Organization-Specific Negative Risks:

    a. _____

    b. _____

    c. _____

V. Action Notes:

☐ Personal Review and Action Chart: Humanistic Standards

1. Rank your own strength in the humanistic standards, on a scale from 1 to 5 (5: very strong, 4: fairly high, 3: adequate, 2: need some improvement, 1: critical).

   Allegiance: _____   Introspection: _____

   Compassion: _____   Spirit: _____

   Dignity: _____

2. Rank the humanistic standards in relative importance to your job (5: vitally important, 4: very important, 3: needed, 2: optional, 1: meaningless).

   Allegiance: _____   Introspection: _____

   Compassion: _____   Spirit: _____

   Dignity: _____

3. Rank your organization's effectiveness in the humanistic standards. (Use the same scale as question #1.)

   Allegiance: _____   Introspection: _____

   Compassion: _____   Spirit: _____

   Dignity: _____

4. Rate your boss relative to the humanistic standards. (Use the same scale as for question #1.)

   Allegiance: _____   Introspection: _____

   Compassion: _____   Spirit: _____

   Dignity: _____

5. List specific positive practical actions you will now undertake:

   a. _____

   b. _____

6. List specific negative counteractions you will try to eliminate:

   a. _____

   b. _____

☐ Business Norms: Standards of Conduct for Fair Business Practices and Ethical Organizational Action

Customer Commitment: Understands that the most important aspect of the health care mission is the provision of top-notch care to the customer and embraces that tenet as a top priority in all work-related activities; realizes that the customer is at the top of the organizational chart in all premier health care organizations.

Forthright Tactics: Employs business standards, sound methods, and solid approaches to all assigned job duties and organizational responsibilities; is as concerned with the "means" of a given assignment as with the end result.

Professional Liberty: Allows each member of the reporting staff to practice his or her trade in an environment of independence and encouragement; motivates individual team members to attain a high degree of professional acumen and a superlative level of competence and confidence.

Quality: Seeks to apply the highest possible quality standards to all work performed by self and all subordinates; is intolerant of needless waste of resources, second-rate effort, or inferior caliber of work production and customer/patient service.

Social Awareness: Possesses an educated frame of reference concerning major social issues that affect the overall health care business; has specific, creditable knowledge of the key sociological issues that affect the organization's local customer population.

☐ Business Norms

Customer Commitment

Understands that the most important aspect of the health care mission is the provision of top-notch care to the customer and embraces that tenet as a top priority in all work-related activities; realizes that the customer is at the top of the organizational chart in all premier health care organizations.

Positive Practical Actions:

- Determines the effect of all work activity on the delivery of customer/patient service
- Seeks information on the needs and desires of customers as related to his or her particular aspect of the business
- Recognizes that the customer drives the organization, not vice-versa
- Instills a respect for and dedication to customer/patient service in all staff members
- Realizes that certain organizational components are "internal customers" and adapts action to assist their efforts
- Supports organizationwide customer relations activities fully through action and key contributions
- Is cognizant of the effect of all pertinent business actions on customer/patient interaction and overall service

Negative Counteractions:

- Perceives individual responsibility as independent and removed from customer service
- Fails to educate staff members on the need of customer/patient awareness
- Is ignorant as to the particular needs and nuances of the organization's customer/patient
- Counteracts organizational customer/patient service programs
- Lacks a general dedication to team effort
- Resents or is biased toward a particular segment of the customer population

☐ Cue Sheet: Business Norms

Customer Commitment

Cue #1: Define *customer commitment* as it relates to the health care organization.

Clues: a. _____

b. _____

Cue #2: How do you instill a sense of customer commitment in your staff?

Clues: a. _____

b. _____

Cue #3: Tell about an employee who particularly exemplified a true sense of customer commitment.

Clues: a. _____

b. _____

Cue #4: How does customer commitment relate specifically to your area(s) of responsibility/technical expertise?

Clues: a. _____

b. _____

Cue #5: What innovations in customer service do you believe to be particularly effective?

Clues: a. _____

b. _____

☐ Progressive Management Factors Work Sheet: Business Norms

Customer Commitment: Understands that the most important aspect of the health care mission is the provision of top-notch care to the customer and embraces that tenet as a top priority in all work-related activities; realizes that the customer is at the top of the organizational chart in all premier health care organizations.

I. Positive Organizational Role Models:

  1. _____

  2. _____

  3. _____

II. Organization-Specific Positive Benefits:

  a. _____

  b. _____

  c. _____

III. Negative Organizational Role Models:

  1. _____

  2. _____

  3. _____

IV. Organization-Specific Negative Risks:

  a. _____

  b. _____

  c. _____

V. Action Notes:

☐ Business Norms

Forthright Tactics

Employs business standards, sound methods, and solid approaches to all assigned job duties and organizational responsibilities; is as concerned with the "means" of a given assignment as with the end result.

Positive Practical Actions:

- Can be depended on to use proper methods in obtaining necessary business results
- Sets an example for coworkers and subordinates in terms of business style
- Never condones questionable methods of operation, even if dramatic financial results can be achieved
- Avoids being sanctimonious or preachy in business approach
- Gets the job done efficiently and effectively, and in a manner that precludes negative repercussions
- Is perceived as being an honest, steady player by all pertinent organizational parties
- Represents the organization well as an ethical, professional health care businessperson

Negative Counteractions:

- Is interested in results to the point that methods are secondary or unimportant
- Uses sound business tactics only when convenient to already-established goals
- Regards ethical tactics as the exception, not the rule, in the perception of staff, superiors, and coworkers
- Stresses results at any cost or method
- Does "little things"—daily actions, backstage activity—that can amount to big trouble
- Has things that constantly "come back to haunt" this individual
- Has work habits that make others apprehensive, nervous, and/or skeptical

☐ Cue Sheet: Business Norms

Forthright Tactics

Cue #1: What constitutes "forthright business tactics" in your estimation?

Clues: a. _____

           b. _____

Cue #2: Is there such a thing as being "too forthright" in business strategy?

Clues: a. _____

           b. _____

Cue #3: Tell about a business situation where utilization of forthright tactics was paramount to success.

Clues: a. _____

           b. _____

Cue #4: Describe an organization you're familiar with that has a well-earned reputation for using forthright business tactics.

Clues: a. _____

           b. _____

Cue #5: Give an example of a situation where you had to "clean up a mess" created by questionable (unethical) business tactics.

Clues: a. _____

           b. _____

☐ Progressive Management Factors Work Sheet: Business Norms

Forthright Tactics: Employs business standards, sound methods, and solid approaches to all assigned job duties and organizational responsibilities; is as concerned with the "means" of a given assignment as with the end result.

  I. Positive Organizational Role Models:

      1. _____

      2. _____

      3. _____

  II. Organization-Specific Positive Benefits:

      a. _____

      b. _____

      c. _____

  III. Negative Organizational Role Models:

      1. _____

      2. _____

      3. _____

  IV. Organization-Specific Negative Risks:

      a. _____

      b. _____

      c. _____

  V. Action Notes:

☐ Business Norms

Professional Liberty

Allows each member of the reporting staff to practice his or her trade in an environment of independence and encouragement; motivates individual team members to attain a high degree of professional acumen and a superlative level of competence and confidence.

Positive Practical Actions:

- Uses delegation skills as appropriately and effectively as possible
- Recognizes the individual skills and talents of each staff member
- Works smoothly with professionals from other departments in matrix management situations
- Optimizes every opportunity to hone the skills of respective subordinates and assist them in reaching their highest professional potential
- Perceives situations where help is needed and skillfully renders that assistance personally or by direction
- Helps staff members address areas of professional weakness and encourages action that will build confidence and strength in key areas
- Leaves individuals to function autonomously and without undue interference or overdirection

Negative Counteractions:

- Constantly questions the competency of subordinates directly or indirectly through actions
- Never permits staff suggestions or alternative methods of addressing a business challenge
- Insults staff members openly by being overcritical and/or demeaning work output
- Lacks tact in discussing various employee weaknesses
- Meddles in projects that are the responsibility of staff members
- Takes undeserved credit for employee achievement

☐ Cue Sheet: Business Norms

Professional Liberty

Cue #1: How much professional liberty should each of your employees have?

Clues: a. _____

b. _____

Cue #2: How would you describe your current reporting staff?

Clues: a. _____

b. _____

Cue #3: What approaches do you take to encourage individual employee growth and professional development?

Clues: a. _____

b. _____

Cue #4: Describe a boss who gave you the ideal degree of professional liberty/latitude/room to grow.

Clues: a. _____

b. _____

Cue #5: Explain the importance of professional liberty/latitude for health care employees.

Clues: a. _____

b. _____

☐ Progressive Management Factors Work Sheet: Business Norms

Professional Liberty: Allows each member of the reporting staff to practice his or her trade in an environment of independence and encouragement; motivates individual team members to attain a high degree of professional acumen and a superlative level of competence and confidence.

I. Positive Organizational Role Models:

　　1. _____

　　2. _____

　　3. _____

II. Organization-Specific Positive Benefits:

　　a. _____

　　b. _____

　　c. _____

III. Negative Organizational Role Models:

　　1. _____

　　2. _____

　　3. _____

IV. Organization-Specific Negative Risks:

　　a. _____

　　b. _____

　　c. _____

V. Action Notes:

☐ Business Norms

Quality

Seeks to apply the highest possible quality standards to all work performed by self and all subordinates; is intolerant of needless waste of resources, second-rate effort, or inferior caliber of work production and customer/patient service.

Positive Practical Actions:

- Sets standards of high quality on performance goals and evaluations
- Initiates and supports quality control and assurance programs throughout the organization
- Produces top-shelf reports, presentations, and other individual work output
- Understands that commitment to quality is not a fad but a daily health care mandate
- Realizes that the quality differential in a successful health care organization can spell the difference between overall success or failure
- Does not abide shortcuts or quick fixes; is willing to take the more difficult but more solid road to successful action
- Condemns shortchanging the customer/patient in terms of service, level of care, and detailed attention
- Takes time to check not only the results of subordinates' action but also their methods and practices

Negative Counteractions:

- Pays only lip service to quality programs and philosophies
- Looks for the quickest, as opposed to the most effective, route to an action conclusion
- Places priority on quantity (numbers) as opposed to quality indicators
- Uses standards of quality selectively; attains a high level on some projects, sinks to a low level on other facets of work role
- Does not provide quality input at meetings, produces shoddy reports, and/or provides inaccurate or nebulous information on key business issues

☐ Cue Sheet: Business Norms

Quality

Cue #1: *Quality,* unfortunately, has become almost a trite expression in health care. What does it mean to you/your job?

Clues: a. _____

b. _____

Cue #2: What quality measures do you use in your professional role?

Clues: a. _____

b. _____

Cue #3: How do you ensure that your work section/department/ employees put quality at the top of their list of work priorities?

Clues: a. _____

b. _____

Cue #4: Describe a health care organization you know that really lives up to high standards of quality.

Clues: a. _____

b. _____

Cue #5: Have you seen situations where only a casual commitment to quality resulted in performance problems? [The interviewer should try to elicit a description of at least one situation.]

Clues: a. _____

b. _____

☐ Progressive Management Factors Work Sheet: Business Norms

Quality: Seeks to apply the highest possible quality standards to all work performed by self and all subordinates; is intolerant of needless waste of resources, second-rate effort, or inferior caliber of work production and customer/patient service.

I. Positive Organizational Role Models:

    1. _____

    2. _____

    3. _____

II. Organization-Specific Positive Benefits:

    a. _____

    b. _____

    c. _____

III. Negative Organizational Role Models:

    1. _____

    2. _____

    3. _____

IV. Organization-Specific Negative Risks:

    a. _____

    b. _____

    c. _____

V. Action Notes:

☐ Business Norms

Social Awareness

Possesses an educated frame of reference concerning major social issues that affect the overall health care business; has specific, creditable knowledge of the key sociological issues that affect the organization's local customer population.

Positive Practical Actions:

- Seeks information from a variety of sources on the key sociological issues related to the delivery of health care services
- Stays in touch with key sociological dimensions of the customer community
- Goes beyond demographics in the quest for pertinent information
- Can anticipate trends that will affect the future delivery of health care services to the customer community
- Has a true, demonstrated compassion for sociological issues that affect both the customer community and segments of the employee population
- Uses the practical relevance of local social issues as part of a comprehensive employee relations program
- Incorporates national social issues into appropriate strategy in both customer service and employee relations

Negative Counteractions:

- Professes feigned ignorance of significant social issues
- Possesses true ignorance toward local social issues
- Has a limited knowledge base of key social issues
- Refuses to correlate key social dynamics to business issues when such action is needed but potentially unpopular
- Never considers social issues to be important business issues
- Is inconsiderate of the sociological and/or ethnic background of employees, as evidenced by words and actions
- Avoids discussing key social issues as they arise; does so only from a reactionary stance

☐ Cue Sheet: Business Norms

Social Awareness

Cue #1: Why is social awareness critical to a health care organization's success?

Clues: a. _____

b. _____

Cue #2: Give an example of a current social issue (local or national) that affects or could affect your job/organization.

Clues: a. _____

b. _____

Cue #3: Define *social awareness* as it relates to health care business.

Clues: a. _____

b. _____

Cue #4: Describe a situation in which your knowledge of social issues promoted business success.

Clues: a. _____

b. _____

Cue #5: How does a sound social awareness fit into your everyday activities?

Clues: a. _____

b. _____

☐ Progressive Management Factors Work Sheet: Business Norms

Social Awareness: Possesses an educated frame of reference concerning major social issues that affect the overall health care business; has specific, creditable knowledge of the key sociological issues that affect the organization's local customer population.

I. Positive Organizational Role Models:

    1. _____

    2. _____

    3. _____

II. Organization-Specific Positive Benefits:

    a. _____

    b. _____

    c. _____

III. Negative Organizational Role Models:

    1. _____

    2. _____

    3. _____

IV. Organization-Specific Negative Risks:

    a. _____

    b. _____

    c. _____

V. Action Notes:

☐ Personal Review and Action Chart: Business Norms

1. Rank your own strength in the business norms, on a scale from 1 to 5 (5: very strong, 4: fairly high, 3: adequate, 2: need some improvement, 1: critical).

   Customer Commitment: _____   Quality: _____

   Forthright Tactics: _____   Social Awareness: _____

   Professional Liberty: _____

2. Rank the business norms in relative importance to your job (5: vitally important, 4: very important, 3: needed, 2: optional, 1: meaningless).

   Customer Commitment: _____   Quality: _____

   Forthright Tactics: _____   Social Awareness: _____

   Professional Liberty: _____

3. Rank your organization's effectiveness in the business norms. (Use the same scale as for question #1.)

   Customer Commitment: _____   Quality: _____

   Forthright Tactics: _____   Social Awareness: _____

   Professional Liberty: _____

4. Rate your boss relative to the business norms. (Use the same scale as for question #1.)

   Customer Commitment: _____   Quality: _____

   Forthright Tactics: _____   Social Awareness: _____

   Professional Liberty: _____

5. List specific positive practical actions you will now undertake:

   a. _____

   b. _____

6. List specific negative counteractions you will try to eliminate:

   a. _____

   b. _____

☐ Executive Principles: Ethical Standards for Leadership Tactics, Organizational Strategy, and Managerial Conduct

Dependability: Makes executive decisions, takes leadership action, and sets organizational policies and standards that are consistent with the attainment of ethical excellence in the provision of high-quality health care services.

Exemplary Conduct: Maintains an organizational leadership role and community presence that reflect a humanistic commitment, positive outlook, and creditable desire to provide stellar service to those in need.

Optimization of Resources: Utilizes all available financial, operational, and human resources to their utmost potential in the interest of efficiency and organizational effectiveness; employs a leadership style that encourages maximum contribution from all organizational members.

Positive Power: Uses the offices of leadership as a charter to serve others and the customer community by displaying competency of management and a spirit of true professionalism in every business endeavor; never abuses power or ignores responsibility in fulfilling executive charter.

Visibility: Steadily maintains a positive "high profile"; always makes leadership and commitment to organizational mission apparent by actions and presence in all business situations, particularly in tough circumstances.

☐ Executive Principles

Dependability

Makes executive decisions, takes leadership action, and sets organizational policies and standards that are consistent with the attainment of ethical excellence in the provision of high-quality health care services.

Positive Practical Actions:

- Can be relied on to consider all viable viewpoints prior to making a decision
- Maintains a sense of continuity from one related action to another
- Is described by most organizational and community members as "consistent," "responsible," or "steady"
- Exhibits dependability that does not become harmful predictability
- Does not waver unnecessarily in making a decision or retract important policy statements
- Has a good frame of reference on most operational aspects of the organization that assists in making quick but effective decisions
- Is seldom second-guessed or criticized when making decisions; makes decisions with suitable knowledge and appropriate force

Negative Counteractions:

- Is often emotional in decision making
- Does not always weigh both sides of a significant issue prior to taking action or making a critical decision
- Makes questionable decisions
- Lets others make decisions that he or she should be making
- Takes the quickest road as opposed to the best road to solving a dilemma
- Is consistent in decision making only if the choice is easy
- Considers ethical action only secondarily in decision making
- Has predictable actions to the extent that quality of leadership is weakened by staff manipulation

☐ Cue Sheet: Executive Principles

Dependability

Cue #1:   What main responsibilities does a health care executive have
          to the organization?

Clues: a. _____

          b. _____

Cue #2:   Define *dependability* as it relates to a health care executive.

Clues: a. _____

          b. _____

Cue #3:   Define *dependability* as it relates to reporting managers on your
          staff.

Clues: a. _____

          b. _____

Cue #4:   What factors go into your decision-making process?

Clues: a. _____

          b. _____

Cue #5:   Describe a situation in which you had to take corrective action
          due to a poor decision.

Clues: a. _____

          b. _____

☐ Progressive Management Factors Work Sheet: Executive Principles

Dependability: Makes executive decisions, takes leadership action, and sets organizational policies and standards that are consistent with the attainment of ethical excellence in the provision of high-quality health care services.

I. Positive Organizational Role Models:

1. _____

2. _____

3. _____

II. Organization-Specific Positive Benefits:

a. _____

b. _____

c. _____

III. Negative Organizational Role Models:

1. _____

2. _____

3. _____

IV. Organization-Specific Negative Risks:

a. _____

b. _____

c. _____

V. Action Notes:

☐ Executive Principles

Exemplary Conduct

Maintains an organizational leadership role and community presence that reflect a humanistic commitment, positive outlook, and creditable desire to provide stellar service to those in need.

Positive Practical Actions:

- Exhibits personal conduct that serves as an example for all organizational members
- Is perceived as being a good person as well as a competent executive
- Has exemplary conduct on and off the job; conduct does not lend itself to being good gossip material
- Demands high ethical standards in the conduct of staff without overstepping boundaries of personal life/professional responsibilities
- Does not impose beliefs on others that are not work related
- Exhibits daily conduct and decision making that consistently represent sound values and solid business ethics
- Can be depended on for strong ethical leadership and personal strength in the face of adversity

Negative Counteractions:

- Exhibits inconsistent personal conduct both on and off the job that is noted by organizational and community members
- Maintains noted high standards on the job but notorious standards off the job
- Inflicts personal standards on organizational members that are not work related
- Exhibits leadership that is suspect in staff's opinion due to inconsistency, lack of values, or overbearing stewardship
- Exhibits conduct in terms of ethics that becomes particularly questionable when the "going gets tough"
- Fails to understand the role of the health care administrator as a high-profile city leader

☐ Cue Sheet: Executive Principles

Exemplary Conduct

Cue #1: What constitutes exemplary conduct by a health care executive?

Clues: a. _____

b. _____

Cue #2: What professional conduct do you expect from your reporting supervisors?

Clues: a. _____

b. _____

Cue #3: Describe an executive you worked with or for or one who worked for you who truly personified exemplary conduct.

Clues: a. _____

b. _____

Cue #4: Has the term *exemplary conduct* (relative to an executive) become a cliché? Why or why not?

Clues: a. _____

b. _____

Cue #5: What type(s) of example(s) should an executive present?

Clues: a. _____

b. _____

☐ Progressive Management Factors Work Sheet: Executive Principles

Exemplary Conduct: Maintains an organizational leadership role and community presence that reflect a humanistic commitment, positive outlook, and creditable desire to provide stellar service to those in need.

I. Positive Organizational Role Models:

    1. _____

    2. _____

    3. _____

II. Organization-Specific Positive Benefits:

    a. _____

    b. _____

    c. _____

III. Negative Organizational Role Models:

    1. _____

    2. _____

    3. _____

IV. Organization-Specific Negative Risks:

    a. _____

    b. _____

    c. _____

V. Action Notes:

☐ Executive Principles

Optimization of Resources

Utilizes all available financial, operational, and human resources to their utmost potential in the interest of efficiency and organizational effectiveness; employs a leadership style that encourages maximum contribution from all organizational members.

Positive Practical Actions:

- Understands the technical strengths of all organizational players
- Never wastes resources unnecessarily
- Considers *efficiency of action* as well as *effectiveness of outcome*
- Is enterprising in using available resources
- Refuses to be intimidated or threatened by lack of an ideal supply of resources
- Understands that human resources are the most important to the organization and often the most challenging to manage
- Seeks to make optimum use of the various resources at hand
- Does not dwell disproportionately on financial resources (or lack of money)

Negative Counteractions:

- Is not fully aware of the ability and potential of organizational members
- Focuses on results at the expense of wasted or over used resources
- Spends unnecessary time worrying about lack of resources as opposed to creative use of resources at hand
- Always gravitates to one facet of resources utilization without full consideration of the "big picture" or to other resources available for task accomplishment
- Will use one person or one resources strategy to the point of overuse/burnout
- Lacks commitment to creative resources utilization
- Wastes resources often due to lack of consideration, understanding, creativity, or commitment

☐ Cue Sheet: Executive Principles

Optimization of Resources

Cue #1: Give an example of a manager who fully utilized all of his or her available resources in getting a job accomplished.

Clues: a. _____

b. _____

Cue #2: Describe a situation in which you had to accomplish a difficult goal with limited resources.

Clues: a. _____

b. _____

Cue #3: Explain the importance of full optimization of resources in the health care workplace.

Clues: a. _____

b. _____

Cue #4: How do you encourage your reporting staff to fully optimize all of their available resources?

Clues: a. _____

b. _____

Cue #5: What problems are inherent in a management scheme where available resources are not used fully?

Clues: a. _____

b. _____

☐ Progressive Management Factors Work Sheet: Executive Principles

Optimization of Resources: Utilizes all available financial, operational, and human resources to their utmost potential in the interest of efficiency and organizational effectiveness; employs a leadership style that encourages maximum contribution from all organizational members.

I. Positive Organizational Role Models:

    1. _____

    2. _____

    3. _____

II. Organization-Specific Positive Benefits:

    a. _____

    b. _____

    c. _____

III. Negative Organizational Role Models:

    1. _____

    2. _____

    3. _____

IV. Organization-Specific Negative Risks:

    a. _____

    b. _____

    c. _____

V. Action Notes:

☐ Executive Principles

Positive Power

Uses the offices of leadership as a charter to serve others and the customer community by displaying competency of management and a spirit of true professionalism in every business endeavor; never abuses power or ignores responsibility in fulfilling executive charter.

Positive Practical Actions:

- Exercises a good balance between power and humility
- Has a clear vision of what the organization is about and what it should accomplish both long term and short term
- Can motivate 10 different staff members in 10 different ways
- Does not let power go to his or her head in any circumstances or situations
- Does not use power to promote favoritism or prejudice
- Is competent in every area of responsibility, from technical aspects to fiscal control to people management
- Is self-demanding in all aspects of the job, which encourages the same spirit of commitment from others
- Uses power to formulate meaningful strategy and ethical tactics

Negative Counteractions:

- Power is abused, as evidenced by:
  - Playing favorites
  - Making unwarranted decisions
  - Undercutting the authority of others
  - Seizing an inordinate number of personal "perks"
  - Lacking a true vision of health care organizational excellence
  - Mismanaging resources, particularly finances
- Uses power as an ax to wield to threaten and manipulate staff members
- Uses power unethically in relation to providing response to community needs
- Is perceived as an autocratic personality
- Uses power unethically, which creates organizational resentment and quashes motivation

☐ Cue Sheet: Executive Principles

Positive Power

Cue #1: What organizational liabilities are incurred by an executive who abuses power?

Clues: a. _____

b. _____

Cue #2: What constitutes abuse of power by a health care executive? [The interviewer should try to elicit examples.]

Clues: a. _____

b. _____

Cue #3: Define *positive executive power.*

Clues: a. _____

b. _____

Cue #4: *Empowerment* is a popular term. What does it mean to you?

Clues: a. _____

b. _____

Cue #5: How does positive power fit into your executive management style?

Clues: a. _____

b. _____

☐ Progressive Management Factors Work Sheet: Executive Principles

Positive Power: Uses the offices of leadership as a charter to serve others and the customer community by displaying competency of management and a spirit of true professionalism in every business endeavor; never abuses power or ignores responsibility in fulfilling executive charter.

I. Positive Organizational Role Models:

    1. _____

    2. _____

    3. _____

II. Organization-Specific Positive Benefits:

    a. _____

    b. _____

    c. _____

III. Negative Organizational Role Models:

    1. _____

    2. _____

    3. _____

IV. Organization-Specific Negative Risks:

    a. _____

    b. _____

    c. _____

V. Action Notes:

☐ Executive Principles

Visibility

Steadily maintains a positive "high profile"; always makes leadership and commitment to organizational mission apparent by actions and presence in all business situations, particularly in tough circumstances.

Positive Practical Actions:

- Presents useful ideas based on sound concepts of health care management whenever participating in meetings and conferences
- Explains the rationale behind tough decisions
- Innovates solid solutions to difficult organizational challenges
- Does not allow executive presence to become domineering or dictatorial
- Supports ethical action by subordinates in a clear, unmistakable manner
- Lets people know his or her position on major issues; leaves nothing to conjecture or guesswork
- Is perceived widely by members of the organization as someone who can be counted on to "do the right thing" in any given business situation
- Increases strength of visibility in dire circumstances so as to support staff who are taking proper actions on behalf of the organization

Negative Counteractions:

- Is nowhere to be found when things get tough
- Never educates appropriate players on why a specific action was taken or a certain position was advocated
- Is always around to take the cheers, never around to hear the boos
- Leaves the responsibility for communicating bad news to subordinates; assumes the responsibility for communicating the good news
- Is rarely accessible to various staff members
- Is virtually a nonentity in the minds of hourly staff and nonexecutive players
- Allows the charter of the organization to be unclear because of his or her lack of accountability and visibility

☐ Cue Sheet: Executive Principles

Visibility

Cue #1: What type of visibility in a position are you most comfortable with?

Clues: a. _____

         b. _____

Cue #2: How does lack of suitable visibility hinder an executive's effectiveness?

Clues: a. _____

         b. _____

Cue #3: Describe an executive you worked with or for who had the proper approach to maintaining creditable visibility.

Clues: a. _____

         b. _____

Cue #4: What role do you usually play in meetings?

Clues: a. _____

         b. _____

Cue #5: How would you depict your executive style?

Clues: a. _____

         b. _____

☐ Progressive Management Factors Work Sheet: Executive Principles

Visibility: Steadily maintains a positive "high profile"; always makes leadership and commitment to organizational mission apparent by actions and presence in all business situations, particularly in tough circumstances.

I. Positive Organizational Role Models:

    1. _____

    2. _____

    3. _____

II. Organization-Specific Positive Benefits:

    a. _____

    b. _____

    c. _____

III. Negative Organizational Role Models:

    1. _____

    2. _____

    3. _____

IV. Organization-Specific Negative Risks:

    a. _____

    b. _____

    c. _____

V. Action Notes:

☐ Personal Review and Action Chart: Executive Principles

1. Rank your own strength in the executive principles, on a scale from 1 to 5 (5: very strong, 4: fairly high, 3: adequate, 2: need some improvement, 1: critical).

   Dependability: _____   Positive Power: _____

   Exemplary Conduct: _____   Visibility: _____

   Optimization of Resources: _____

2. Rank the executive principles in relative importance to your job (5: vitally important, 4: very important, 3: needed, 2: optional, 1: meaningless).

   Dependability: _____   Positive Power: _____

   Exemplary Conduct: _____   Visibility: _____

   Optimization of Resources: _____

3. Rank your organization's effectiveness in the executive principles. (Use the same scale as for question #1.)

   Dependability: _____   Positive Power: _____

   Exemplary Conduct: _____   Visibility: _____

   Optimization of Resources: _____

4. Rate your boss relative to the executive principles. (Use the same scale as for question #1.)

   Dependability: _____   Positive Power: _____

   Exemplary Conduct: _____   Visibility: _____

   Optimization of Resources: _____

5. List specific positive practical actions you will now undertake:

   a. _____

   b. _____

6. List specific negative counteractions you will try to eliminate:

   a. _____

   b. _____

Value-Driven Performance Evaluation Plan

As discussed throughout this book, the use of a value-driven approach to performance management mandates a strategy for numerically scoring performance relative to the organization's performance values. This appendix offers a scheme for rating not only an employee's performance toward specific goals based on the job description, but also the degree of employee commitment to desirable personal values, humanistic standards, business norms, and executive principles.

The format can be modified to an organization's current performance evaluation system, or it can be used as the basis for a new, more comprehensive one. Furthermore, it works in concert with the personnel development planning process (chapters 7 and 8) and other approaches to progressive management detailed in this book.

Some approaches that should be considered as an organization tailors the evaluation system for its use include:

- Adding, deleting, or substituting the most important value factors in section II as the organization deems appropriate
- Utilizing the significant actions/critical contributions form in section III for all employees
- Using the performance evaluation planning forms on a new employee's first day as a guidance tool

☐ Section I. Evaluation of Duties, Responsibilities, Goals, and Objectives

Using the employee's job description as well as the goals and objectives set at the beginning of the review period, the reviewing manager should first determine up to 10 factors on which to evaluate the employee's significant overall performance.

Duties are factors in the employee's job description that are ongoing in nature and vital to consistently good standards of performance.

Responsibilities are also drawn from the job description and are facets of the job that can be evaluated quantitatively in terms of numerical increases/decreases, percentage increases/decreases, cost reductions, time reductions, and other clearly defined representations of job performance.

Goals are broad activities and efforts assigned by the reviewing manager at the beginning of the review period that can reflect significant improvements in performance when compared with a previous review period.

Objectives are specific actions that have been agreed to by the reviewer and the employee at the beginning of the review period and that represent measurable gains in the effectiveness of quality and/or efficiency of the employee's performance.

At the beginning of the review period, the reviewing manager should establish the factors to be evaluated in this section, using both the job description as well as the manager's familiarity with the critical needs of the work position. It is recommended that the total number of factors in this section not exceed 10 items, because the factors should be representative of the *major* facets of the employee's performance. Each factor must have a weighted value attached to it, using multiples of 5 points and contributing to a total of 100 points for section I.

In performing the evaluation at the end of the review period on the accompanying grid, each factor should be coded according to a 1–3-point scale as follows:

1 Below expectations: Substandard performance as it relates to the assigned work factor

2 Meets expectations: Satisfactory performance as it relates to the assigned work factor

3 Exceeds expectations: Outstanding performance as it relates to the assigned work factor

After assigning the code for each factor using this scale, multiply the code by the number of points assigned to the factor. This yields the performance score. Brief comments pertaining to performance with regard to that factor should be written alongside the score and are required for codes of 1 or 3. A final total for all the performance scores in section I should be computed and recorded at the bottom of the accompanying grid. The maximum total score is 300.

In establishing the evaluation factors in section I, and in collecting evidence, the reviewing manager must be certain to refer to his or her institution's employee handbook and any other related guidance. The manager should also be sure to periodically review the employee's progress throughout the year by referring back to the established evaluation factors, preferably at least once every three months, in order to ensure successful adherence to good standards of performance.

☐ Section I (Continued). Performance Factors Evaluation Grid

Performance Evaluation Factor	Weighted Value (Points)	Code	Performance Score	Comments
1.				
2.				
3.				
4.				
5.				
6.				
7.				
8.				
9.				
10.				
Total Performance Score				

☐ Section II. Evaluation of Performance Values

The work conduct of the organization's employees—as it pertains to the organization's mission, philosophy, and objectives—is vitally important to the long-term success of the organization. In section II, the reviewing manager evaluates 20 performance values to ascertain the degree to which employees demonstrate these values in their work lives.

Section II values, which are listed and defined on the accompanying grid, should be rated according to a 1–5-point scale:

1 Poor performance: Must be corrected immediately to retain employment

2 Marginal performance: Must be corrected within the next rating period

3 Satisfactory performance: No improvement mandated but performance should nevertheless be enhanced

4 Good performance: Employee is one of the best performers in the rating group

5 Exemplary performance: Employee is the absolute best performer in the rating group

The total number of values, multiplied by the top number of points available for each value (that is, 5), allows for a maximum total of 100 points. The employee's total should be computed and recorded. Any value scored as a 1 or a 5 must be documented appropriately in the "Relevance to Job Conduct" space provided on the accompanying grid.

☐ Section II (Continued). Performance Values Evaluation Grid

Personal Values

Performance Value	Points	Relevance to Job Conduct
Decency Consistently demonstrates a basic sense of propriety as it applies to the human factor in the workplace; never places the desire to "do the right thing" in a secondary role in the workplace.		
Fortitude Brings a sound, unpretentious quality of courage to the everyday workplace that enables the capacity to make tough decisions and seek the most ethical solution to any business challenge; is patient in obtaining solid results and steadfast in constructing ethically optimum plans.		
Industry Understands the need to dedicate one's efforts to maximum effectiveness and efficiency every day and in all business circumstances; readily accepts the daily responsibility of being a role model of quality output and optimum effort and production.		
Integrity Incorporates honor, truthfulness, and sincerity into an everyday work philosophy; is uncompromising in seeking		

Personal Values

Performance Value	Points	Relevance to Job Conduct
the factual evidence in every situation and resolute in providing upright stances and credible data in all situations.		
Knowledge Constantly pursues growth and development activities that strengthen business knowledge, technical acumen, and personal enhancement; realizes that there is something to be learned every day and in every situation, and that attainment of as much knowledge as possible is a responsibility and requirement of ethical leadership.		

Humanistic Standards

Performance Value	Points	Relevance to Job Conduct
Allegiance Demonstrates through words and actions a fidelity to helping those in need and supporting others engaged in the provision of superior health care; is unwavering in assisting those in need and giving maximum effort in both individual and group activities that benefit the organization.		
Compassion Sensitivity toward others is reflected in acceptance of varied personalities,		

Humanistic Standards

Performance Value	Points	Relevance to Job Conduct
appreciation of cultural differences, and a genuine affection for people that transcends clichés and superficial statements and is expressed in continuous action both on and off the job.		
Dignity Provides all employees the opportunity to grow and develop full professional potential; respects every employee and promotes a workplace climate where each professional is treated as the most important asset.		
Introspection Constantly challenges self to attain the highest degree of professional achievement and maintain the best ethical standards in all situations; is consistent in thinking through important issues, balancing consequences with action, and tempering firmness with humanistic consideration.		
Spirit Manifests a self-generated positive attitude toward the health care industry, a vitality toward everyday responsibilities, and an incessant desire to become a better professional and person; has an infectious enthusiasm for the health care workplace and its important mission.		

Business Norms

Performance Value	Points	Relevance to Job Conduct
Customer Commitment Understands that the most important aspect of the health care mission is the provision of top-notch care to the customer and embraces that tenet as a top priority in all work-related activities; realizes that the customer is at the top of the organizational chart in all premier health care organizations.		
Forthright Tactics Employs business standards, sound methods, and solid approaches to all assigned job duties and organizational responsibilities; is as concerned with the "means" of a given assignment as with the end result.		
Professional Liberty Allows each member of the reporting staff to practice his or her trade in an environment of independence and encouragement; motivates individual team members to attain a high degree of professional acumen and a superlative level of competence and confidence.		
Quality Seeks to apply the highest possible quality standards to all work performed by self and all subordinates;		

Business Norms

Performance Value	Points	Relevance to Job Conduct
is intolerant of needless waste of resources, second-rate effort, or inferior caliber of work production and customer/patient service.		
Social Awareness Possesses an educated frame of reference concerning major social issues that affect the overall health care business; has specific, creditable knowledge of the key sociological issues that affect the organization's local customer population.		

Executive Principles

Performance Value	Points	Relevance to Job Conduct
Dependability Makes executive decisions, takes leadership action, and sets organizational policies and standards that are consistent with the attainment of ethical excellence in the provision of high-quality health care services.		
Exemplary Conduct Maintains an organizational leadership role and community presence that reflects a humanistic commitment, positive outlook and creditable desire to provide stellar service to those in need.		

Executive Principles

Performance Value	Points	Relevance to Job Conduct
Optimization of Resources Utilizes all available financial, operational, and human resources to their utmost potential in the interest of efficiency and organizational effectiveness; employs a leadership style that encourages maximum contribution from all organizational members.		
Positive Power Uses the offices of leadership as a charter to serve others and the customer community by displaying competency of management and a spirit of true professionalism in every business endeavor; never abuses power or ignores responsibility in fulfilling executive charter.		
Visibility Steadily maintains a positive "high profile"; always makes leadership and commitment to organizational mission apparent by actions and presence in all business situations, particularly in tough circumstances.		
Total Points		

☐ Section III. Evaluation of Significant Actions/Critical Contributions

This section is utilized to cite performance that is special in nature and is not reflected in the evaluation in Section I. The first column of the accompanying grid is used to describe any significant actions or critical contributions to the organization made by the employee during the rating period.

The second column, labeled "Code," is for assigning a performance category. The 12 possible performance categories and their code letters are:

a. Performance that is clearly "above and beyond the call of duty" in which the employee responded in a stellar fashion. If a crisis occurred and the employee responded negatively, this should be cited on the evaluation grid *but not given any points at all.*

b. A major cost-saving program instituted and proved efficient, as evidenced by significant budget numbers.

c. New program implementation, where the employee designed and implemented a program that provided a major, measurable organizational benefit.

d. Time efficiency as produced by a new operational approach, new system, or new program, which substantially improved time effectiveness.

e. Operational improvement, such as a procedure upgrading or practice/system innovation that enhances flow of operation significantly.

f. Major quality improvement that has a marked benefit to users and performers and adds to the organization's overall quality management program.

g. Undertaking of new responsibilities created by unforeseen circumstances, such as turnover, crisis, expansion, and so forth.

h. Productivity enhancements, such as new programs, inventions, innovations, or other creations that spark increased productivity.

i. Human resources maximization, where the employee has devised a new strategy for optimizing the contribution of each relevant employee.

j. Positive reaction to a major, unforeseen negative crisis that taxes the entire work unit. Performer demonstrated quick, effective action and provided leadership by example.

k. Undertaking of a new, major project or program not assigned at the start of the performance review period.

l. Major development activities that increase the employee's professional expertise as well as contribution to the organization.

The third column, labeled "Points Assigned," is for giving each significant action or critical contribution a score using multiples of 5 points. Each 5 points requires at least one code justification. If a crisis occurred and the employee missed an opportunity for a significant action or critical contribution to the organization, or if the employee responded negatively, this opportunity should be cited and given no points on the form.

The reviewing manager must be fair in evaluating each significant action or critical contribution, and must be very circumspect in giving the performer a truly representative grading in terms of points assigned. The total number of points an employee can earn is up to the employee according to his or her individual initiative, though a maximum goal of 100 points is suggested. Obviously, an employee performing *only* the duties outlined in his or her job description would receive no points in section III.

☐ Section III (Continued). Significant Action/Critical Contribution Evaluation Grid

The reviewing manager should cite any reactions to significant incidents and/or any critical contributions made by the employee during the performance rating period, and record the code(s) reflecting the nature of the action(s) or contribution(s), as well as the assigned points, on the following grid. Five points can be assigned for each code at the reviewing manager's discretion, as per the institution's performance evaluation guidelines. Negative reactions to significant incidents should be recorded but assigned no points.

Significant Action/ Critical Contribution	Code	Points Assigned	Comments
1.			
2.			
3.			
4.			
5.			
6.			
7.			
8.			
9.			
10.			
11.			
12.			
13.			
14.			
15.			
16.			
17.			
18.			
19.			
20.			
Total Points			

☐ Appendix C

Progressive Motivational Strategies

As discussed in chapter 4, a wide array of motivational strategies is needed for progressive health care management. This appendix describes 50 motivators in 5 key areas.

Review all of the motivators and, using the work sheets, prepare an enhancement strategy for your reporting staff. A sample work sheet filled out by the author appears in figure C-1.

Figure C-1. Sample Motivator Work Sheet

Achievement: The organization's members are encouraged to aspire and work toward their respective highest level of performance and are provided with the support and resources to reach those levels.

1. Pertinent examples in my organization [both positive and negative]:
   a. D. Flanagan (+)
   b. W. Sharisky (+)
   c. T. Lawrence (−)

2. Potential targets on my reporting staff:
   a. J. Rivers
   b. T. Lawrence
   c. K. D'Angelo

3. Departmental targets within my organization:
   a. Housekeeping
   b. Accounts Payable
   c. Medical Records

4. Applicable enhancement strategies:
   a. Mission achievement committees
   b. Criterion-based performance evaluation
   c. Personnel development planning (PDP) system

5. Notes:
   Reset performance objectives of J. Rivers, T. Lawrence, and K. D'Angelo.
   Establish "bonus for excellence" system in targeted departments.

☐ Environmental and Organization-Driven Motivators

1. Affiliation
2. Corporate Culture Norms
3. Leadership
4. Mission Identification
5. Organizational Design
6. Organizational Development
7. Organizational Direction and Goals
8. Organizational Ethics
9. Organizational Power and Influence
10. Security
11. Social Interaction
12. Stability
13. Tangible Benefits

☐ Environmental and Organization-Driven Motivators

Affiliation: Employees have a sense of belonging, of working with a "winning entity," one that is dedicated to positive action and high-quality service provision.

1. Pertinent examples in my organization:

   a. _____

   b. _____

   c. _____

2. Potential targets on my reporting staff:

   a. _____

   b. _____

   c. _____

3. Department targets within my organization:

   a. _____

   b. _____

   c. _____

4. Applicable enhancement strategies:

   a. _____

   b. _____

   c. _____

5. Notes:

☐ Environment and Organization-Driven Motivators

Corporate Culture Norms: Ethical and organizational personality dimensions are "in sync" with the personal values and work personality of the individual, and encourage maximum output and dedication to group objectives.

1. Pertinent examples in my organization:

   a. _____

   b. _____

   c. _____

2. Potential targets on my reporting staff:

   a. _____

   b. _____

   c. _____

3. Department targets within my organization:

   a. _____

   b. _____

   c. _____

4. Applicable enhancement strategies:

   a. _____

   b. _____

   c. _____

5. Notes:

☐ Environmental and Organization-Driven Motivators

Leadership: There is inspirational direction and clear vision of organizational direction that establish a sense of trust between upper management and all employees as well as long-term employee commitment.

1. Pertinent examples in my organization:

   a. _____

   b. _____

   c. _____

2. Potential targets on my reporting staff:

   a. _____

   b. _____

   c. _____

3. Department targets within my organization:

   a. _____

   b. _____

   c. _____

4. Applicable enhancement strategies:

   a. _____

   b. _____

   c. _____

5. Notes:

☐ Environmental and Organization-Driven Motivators

Mission Identification: Individual employees identify clearly with the overall mission of the organization and its commitment to providing high-quality health care services to a designated community.

1. Pertinent examples in my organization:

    a. _____

    b. _____

    c. _____

2. Potential targets on my reporting staff:

    a. _____

    b. _____

    c. _____

3. Department targets within my organization:

    a. _____

    b. _____

    c. _____

4. Applicable enhancement strategies:

    a. _____

    b. _____

    c. _____

5. Notes:

☐ **Environmental and Organization-Driven Motivators**

Organizational Design: Organizational structure and reporting relationships enable maximum interchange and fluid action, quick response to work requests, and timely approval of necessary action.

1. Pertinent examples in my organization:

    a. _____

    b. _____

    c. _____

2. Potential targets on my reporting staff:

    a. _____

    b. _____

    c. _____

3. Department targets within my organization:

    a. _____

    b. _____

    c. _____

4. Applicable enhancement strategies:

    a. _____

    b. _____

    c. _____

5. Notes:

☐ **Environmental and Organization-Driven Motivators**

Organizational Development: Organizational growth, as evidenced by positive reaction to environmental change and constant upgrading of services and resources, inspires proactive, steady individual performance.

1. Pertinent examples in my organization:

    a. _____

    b. _____

    c. _____

2. Potential targets on my reporting staff:

    a. _____

    b. _____

    c. _____

3. Department targets within my organization:

    a. _____

    b. _____

    c. _____

4. Applicable enhancement strategies:

    a. _____

    b. _____

    c. _____

5. Notes:

☐ **Environmental and Organization-Driven Motivators**

Organizational Direction and Goals: Long-range plans and aspirations of the organization are meaningful to the employee and generate a sense of enthusiasm and progressive action within the work group.

1. Pertinent examples in my organization:

   a. _____

   b. _____

   c. _____

2. Potential targets on my reporting staff:

   a. _____

   b. _____

   c. _____

3. Department targets within my organization:

   a. _____

   b. _____

   c. _____

4. Applicable enhancement strategies:

   a. _____

   b. _____

   c. _____

5. Notes:

☐ **Environmental and Organization-Driven Motivators**

Organizational Ethics: There is adherence throughout the organization to a set of humanistic standards, upright business practices, and organizational values that enhance value-based daily action.

1. Pertinent examples in my organization:

   a. _____

   b. _____

   c. _____

2. Potential targets on my reporting staff:

   a. _____

   b. _____

   c. _____

3. Department targets within my organization:

   a. _____

   b. _____

   c. _____

4. Applicable enhancement strategies:

   a. _____

   b. _____

   c. _____

5. Notes:

□ **Environmental and Organization-Driven Motivators**

Organizational Power and Influence: There is an accurate perception on the part of all employees that their organization is a positive and powerful presence within their competitive environment.

1. Pertinent examples in my organization:

   a. _____

   b. _____

   c. _____

2. Potential targets on my reporting staff:

   a. _____

   b. _____

   c. _____

3. Department targets within my organization:

   a. _____

   b. _____

   c. _____

4. Applicable enhancement strategies:

   a. _____

   b. _____

   c. _____

5. Notes:

☐ Environmental and Organization-Driven Motivators

Security: The organization's fiscal stability and ability to achieve profitability under changing conditions provide a sense of job and income security to all employees.

1. Pertinent examples in my organization:

   a. _____

   b. _____

   c. _____

2. Potential targets on my reporting staff:

   a. _____

   b. _____

   c. _____

3. Department targets within my organization:

   a. _____

   b. _____

   c. _____

4. Applicable enhancement strategies:

   a. _____

   b. _____

   c. _____

5. Notes:

☐ **Environmental and Organization-Driven Motivators**

Social Interaction: There is a basic sense on the part of each employee that coworkers are "my type of people"; that they have a similar commitment to health care, common professional aspirations, and personal values.

1. Pertinent examples in my organization:

   a. _____

   b. _____

   c. _____

2. Potential targets on my reporting staff:

   a. _____

   b. _____

   c. _____

3. Department targets within my organization:

   a. _____

   b. _____

   c. _____

4. Applicable enhancement strategies:

   a. _____

   b. _____

   c. _____

5. Notes:

☐ Environmental and Organization-Driven Motivators

Stability: Turbulent external change does not drastically affect the overall organization, and internal change does not impede individual work roles or personal growth and progress.

1. Pertinent examples in my organization:

   a. _____

   b. _____

   c. _____

2. Potential targets on my reporting staff:

   a. _____

   b. _____

   c. _____

3. Department targets within my organization:

   a. _____

   b. _____

   c. _____

4. Applicable enhancement strategies:

   a. _____

   b. _____

   c. _____

5. Notes:

☐ **Environmental and Organization-Driven Motivators**

Tangible Benefits: There are organizationally generated, measurable advantages of employment, including various forms of insurance, fiscal rewards, educational opportunities, and other incentive-based benefits.

1. Pertinent examples in my organization:

   a. _____

   b. _____

   c. _____

2. Potential targets on my reporting staff:

   a. _____

   b. _____

   c. _____

3. Department targets within my organization:

   a. _____

   b. _____

   c. _____

4. Applicable enhancement strategies:

   a. _____

   b. _____

   c. _____

5. Notes:

☐ Management-Controlled Motivators

1. Achievement
2. Change
3. Fun Quotient
4. Group Orientation and Organization
5. Independence
6. Management Style
7. Recognition
8. Reward Systems
9. Work Interest
10. Workplace Progressive Action

☐ **Management-Controlled Motivators**

Achievement: The organization's members are encouraged to aspire and work toward their respective highest level of performance and are provided with the support and resources to reach those levels.

1. Pertinent examples in my organization:

   a. _____

   b. _____

   c. _____

2. Potential targets on my reporting staff:

   a. _____

   b. _____

   c. _____

3. Department targets within my organization:

   a. _____

   b. _____

   c. _____

4. Applicable enhancement strategies:

   a. _____

   b. _____

   c. _____

5. Notes:

☐ **Management-Controlled Motivators**

Change: Employees and managers respond to new dimensions in the workplace, increased demands for output, shifting objectives, assimilation of new resources, and productive management of altering performance standards and factors.

1. Pertinent examples in my organization:

    a. _____

    b. _____

    c. _____

2. Potential targets on my reporting staff:

    a. _____

    b. _____

    c. _____

3. Department targets within my organization:

    a. _____

    b. _____

    c. _____

4. Applicable enhancement strategies:

    a. _____

    b. _____

    c. _____

5. Notes:

☐ **Management-Controlled Motivators**

Fun Quotient: There is simple enjoyment of the workplace and a majority of its activities, which renews industry on an individual basis and spirit of accomplishment on a group basis.

1. Pertinent examples in my organization:

   a. _____

   b. _____

   c. _____

2. Potential targets on my reporting staff:

   a. _____

   b. _____

   c. _____

3. Department targets within my organization:

   a. _____

   b. _____

   c. _____

4. Applicable enhancement strategies:

   a. _____

   b. _____

   c. _____

5. Notes:

☐ **Management-Controlled Motivators**

Group Orientation and Organization: Work teams are structured for maximum individual contribution and performance aimed toward achieving established organizational and group goals and objectives.

1. Pertinent examples in my organization:

   a. _____

   b. _____

   c. _____

2. Potential targets on my reporting staff:

   a. _____

   b. _____

   c. _____

3. Department targets within my organization:

   a. _____

   b. _____

   c. _____

4. Applicable enhancement strategies:

   a. _____

   b. _____

   c. _____

5. Notes:

☐ **Management-Controlled Motivators**

Independence: There is a relative degree of autonomy given to each employee in the pursuit of set goals and objectives, as well as the degree of input allowed from the employee in setting those goals.

1. Pertinent examples in my organization:

   a. _____

   b. _____

   c. _____

2. Potential targets on my reporting staff:

   a. _____

   b. _____

   c. _____

3. Department targets within my organization:

   a. _____

   b. _____

   c. _____

4. Applicable enhancement strategies:

   a. _____

   b. _____

   c. _____

5. Notes:

☐ Management-Controlled Motivators

Management Style: The method of the organization's control and administration, whether autocratic, pyramid, or participative, is inspirational and encouraging of optimum individual performance.

1. Pertinent examples in my organization:

    a. _____

    b. _____

    c. _____

2. Potential targets on my reporting staff:

    a. _____

    b. _____

    c. _____

3. Department targets within my organization:

    a. _____

    b. _____

    c. _____

4. Applicable enhancement strategies:

    a. _____

    b. _____

    c. _____

5. Notes:

☐ **Management-Controlled Motivators**

Recognition: Methods of publicizing stellar performance throughout the organization are employed in the interest of encouraging maximum performance and inspiring other organizational members to make exemplary contributions through their work efforts.

1. Pertinent examples in my organization:

    a. _____

    b. _____

    c. _____

2. Potential targets on my reporting staff:

    a. _____

    b. _____

    c. _____

3. Department targets within my organization:

    a. _____

    b. _____

    c. _____

4. Applicable enhancement strategies:

    a. _____

    b. _____

    c. _____

5. Notes:

☐ Management-Controlled Motivators

Reward Systems: There are procedures for rewarding outstanding performance that have organizational impact and importance, including monetary and nonmonetary compensation and remuneration.

1. Pertinent examples in my organization:

   a. _____

   b. _____

   c. _____

2. Potential targets on my reporting staff:

   a. _____

   b. _____

   c. _____

3. Department targets within my organization:

   a. _____

   b. _____

   c. _____

4. Applicable enhancement strategies:

   a. _____

   b. _____

   c. _____

5. Notes:

☐ **Management-Controlled Motivators**

Work Interest: There is a genuine affinity for the type of work encompassed by the job position, and the positive exploitation of that interest by management to increase employee performance.

1. Pertinent examples in my organization:

   a. _____

   b. _____

   c. _____

2. Potential targets on my reporting staff:

   a. _____

   b. _____

   c. _____

3. Department targets within my organization:

   a. _____

   b. _____

   c. _____

4. Applicable enhancement strategies:

   a. _____

   b. _____

   c. _____

5. Notes:

☐ **Management-Controlled Motivators**

Workplace Progressive Action: The continuous upgrading of process and regeneration of quality standards are accomplished by the organization and each individual work group on a regular basis.

1. Pertinent examples in my organization:

   a. _____

   b. _____

   c. _____

2. Potential targets on my reporting staff:

   a. _____

   b. _____

   c. _____

3. Department targets within my organization:

   a. _____

   b. _____

   c. _____

4. Applicable enhancement strategies:

   a. _____

   b. _____

   c. _____

5. Notes:

☐ Individual Motivators

1. Authority
2. Decision-Making Power
3. Ego
4. Intangible Benefits
5. Money
6. Personal Growth
7. Satisfaction
8. Supervisory Responsibilities
9. Work Personality

☐ Individual Motivators

Authority: There is a degree of control relegated to an employee relative to job-related power and scope of work responsibility; there also is an individual power base within the overall group scheme.

1. Pertinent examples in my organization:

   a. _____

   b. _____

   c. _____

2. Potential targets on my reporting staff:

   a. _____

   b. _____

   c. _____

3. Department targets within my organization:

   a. _____

   b. _____

   c. _____

4. Applicable enhancement strategies:

   a. _____

   b. _____

   c. _____

5. Notes:

☐ **Individual Motivators**

Decision-Making Power: Employees have latitude to enact programs and enforce policy within a set parameter of organizational responsibility in an independent manner that encourages creativity and accountability.

1. Pertinent examples in my organization:

   a. _____

   b. _____

   c. _____

2. Potential targets on my reporting staff:

   a. _____

   b. _____

   c. _____

3. Department targets within my organization:

   a. _____

   b. _____

   c. _____

4. Applicable enhancement strategies:

   a. _____

   b. _____

   c. _____

5. Notes:

☐ **Individual Motivators**

Ego: Employees bring a certain depth of self-esteem to the workplace and need to have a feeling of self-worth and ego gratification from their progressive work contributions.

1. Pertinent examples in my organization:

    a. _____

    b. _____

    c. _____

2. Potential targets on my reporting staff:

    a. _____

    b. _____

    c. _____

3. Department targets within my organization:

    a. _____

    b. _____

    c. _____

4. Applicable enhancement strategies:

    a. _____

    b. _____

    c. _____

5. Notes:

☐ Individual Motivators

Intangible Benefits: Important, nonmonetary job rewards are provided that are highly valued by the individual and uniquely provided by the organization; these benefits meet a personal need or want, for example, geographic location of the organization.

1. Pertinent examples in my organization:

   a. _____

   b. _____

   c. _____

2. Potential targets on my reporting staff:

   a. _____

   b. _____

   c. _____

3. Department targets within my organization:

   a. _____

   b. _____

   c. _____

4. Applicable enhancement strategies:

   a. _____

   b. _____

   c. _____

5. Notes:

☐ **Individual Motivators**

Money: The level of compensation, principally salary dollars, represents a fair measure of the employee's expertise and overall contribution relative to local job market criteria.

1. Pertinent examples in my organization:

   a. _____

   b. _____

   c. _____

2. Potential targets on my reporting staff:

   a. _____

   b. _____

   c. _____

3. Department targets within my organization:

   a. _____

   b. _____

   c. _____

4. Applicable enhancement strategies:

   a. _____

   b. _____

   c. _____

5. Notes:

☐ Individual Motivators

Personal Growth: Individuals place a premium on the extent of growth provided by the job situation relative to nontechnical, interpersonal, and self-development enhancement.

1. Pertinent examples in my organization:

    a. _____

    b. _____

    c. _____

2. Potential targets on my reporting staff:

    a. _____

    b. _____

    c. _____

3. Department targets within my organization:

    a. _____

    b. _____

    c. _____

4. Applicable enhancement strategies:

    a. _____

    b. _____

    c. _____

5. Notes:

☐ **Individual Motivators**

Satisfaction: Self-fulfillment, as defined by the employee, is reflected by his or her daily contribution to the health care workplace and the knowledge that the contribution is vitally needed.

1. Pertinent examples in my organization:

    a. _____

    b. _____

    c. _____

2. Potential targets on my reporting staff:

    a. _____

    b. _____

    c. _____

3. Department targets within my organization:

    a. _____

    b. _____

    c. _____

4. Applicable enhancement strategies:

    a. _____

    b. _____

    c. _____

5. Notes:

☐ **Individual Motivators**

Supervisory Responsibilities: A level of supervision regarding human resources, operational assignments, equipment, or fiscal resources is delegated to the employee by the organization.

1. Pertinent examples in my organization:

   a. _____

   b. _____

   c. _____

2. Potential targets on my reporting staff:

   a. _____

   b. _____

   c. _____

3. Department targets within my organization:

   a. _____

   b. _____

   c. _____

4. Applicable enhancement strategies:

   a. _____

   b. _____

   c. _____

5. Notes:

☐ **Individual Motivators**

Work Personality: An employee's attitude orientation, people skills and interpersonal strengths, managerial aptitude, and team orientation are encouraged and well placed within the organization.

1. Pertinent examples in my organization:

    a. _____

    b. _____

    c. _____

2. Potential targets on my reporting staff:

    a. _____

    b. _____

    c. _____

3. Department targets within my organization:

    a. _____

    b. _____

    c. _____

4. Applicable enhancement strategies:

    a. _____

    b. _____

    c. _____

5. Notes:

☐ Job-Related Motivators

1. Advancement
2. Communication
3. Enhancement
4. Job Description
5. Job Design
6. Negative Consequences
7. Positive Management of Stress
8. Significant Responsibility
9. Work Climate

☐ Job-Related Motivators

Advancement: Clear opportunities are provided throughout the organization for promotion and new challenge, replete with greater compensation and intangible rewards, and increased and desired responsibility.

1. Pertinent examples in my organization:

   a. _____

   b. _____

   c. _____

2. Potential targets on my reporting staff:

   a. _____

   b. _____

   c. _____

3. Department targets within my organization:

   a. _____

   b. _____

   c. _____

4. Applicable enhancement strategies:

   a. _____

   b. _____

   c. _____

5. Notes:

☐ Job-Related Motivators

Communication: Information is shared appropriately throughout the workplace, adding to the employee's knowledge base and awareness of the "big picture"; this includes clear direction and opportunity for feedback and input.

1. Pertinent examples in my organization:

    a. _____

    b. _____

    c. _____

2. Potential targets on my reporting staff:

    a. _____

    b. _____

    c. _____

3. Department targets within my organization:

    a. _____

    b. _____

    c. _____

4. Applicable enhancement strategies:

    a. _____

    b. _____

    c. _____

5. Notes:

☐ Job-Related Motivators

Enhancement: This is the opportunity for creative expansion of job scope by addition of tasks that are of special interest to the employee and/or take positive advantage of specific skills, and are balanced with appropriate rewards.

1. Pertinent examples in my organization:

    a. _____

    b. _____

    c. _____

2. Potential targets on my reporting staff:

    a. _____

    b. _____

    c. _____

3. Department targets within my organization:

    a. _____

    b. _____

    c. _____

4. Applicable enhancement strategies:

    a. _____

    b. _____

    c. _____

5. Notes:

☐ Job-Related Motivators

Job Description: The major areas of ongoing job activity are documented, including contents of the everyday job activities that comprise the majority (65 percent or more) of compensated performance and evaluated output.

1. Pertinent examples in my organization:

   a. _____

   b. _____

   c. _____

2. Potential targets on my reporting staff:

   a. _____

   b. _____

   c. _____

3. Department targets within my organization:

   a. _____

   b. _____

   c. _____

4. Applicable enhancement strategies:

   a. _____

   b. _____

   c. _____

5. Notes:

☐ Job-Related Motivators

Job Design: The structure of the particular work role is delineated, including lines of report, matrix dimensions, avenues of communication, and allocated resources for task accomplishment and continuous action.

1. Pertinent examples in my organization:

    a. _____

    b. _____

    c. _____

2. Potential targets on my reporting staff:

    a. _____

    b. _____

    c. _____

3. Department targets within my organization:

    a. _____

    b. _____

    c. _____

4. Applicable enhancement strategies:

    a. _____

    b. _____

    c. _____

5. Notes:

☐ Job-Related Motivators

Negative Consequences: Certain actions that must be taken in a timely fashion to avoid pejorative or counteractive outcomes, and certain circumstances must be addressed by positive action to maintain workplace progress.

1. Pertinent examples in my organization:

    a. _____

    b. _____

    c. _____

2. Potential targets on my reporting staff:

    a. _____

    b. _____

    c. _____

3. Department targets within my organization:

    a. _____

    b. _____

    c. _____

4. Applicable enhancement strategies:

    a. _____

    b. _____

    c. _____

5. Notes:

☐ Job-Related Motivators

Positive Management of Stress: Work action is pursued without unnecessary acceleration of pace, undue pressure from management, or outside sources and in an atmosphere where change is managed positively and productively.

1. Pertinent examples in my organization:

   a. _____

   b. _____

   c. _____

2. Potential targets on my reporting staff:

   a. _____

   b. _____

   c. _____

3. Department targets within my organization:

   a. _____

   b. _____

   c. _____

4. Applicable enhancement strategies:

   a. _____

   b. _____

   c. _____

5. Notes:

☐ Job-Related Motivators

Significant Responsibility: Factors of performance are evaluated that are part of the employee's everyday job standards and the ongoing expectations of the organization but are not specified in the job description.

1. Pertinent examples in my organization:

   a. _____

   b. _____

   c. _____

2. Potential targets on my reporting staff:

   a. _____

   b. _____

   c. _____

3. Department targets within my organization:

   a. _____

   b. _____

   c. _____

4. Applicable enhancement strategies:

   a. _____

   b. _____

   c. _____

5. Notes:

☐ Job-Related Motivators

Work Climate: Combined physical environmental factors (such as lighting, desk space, and noise control) and psychological factors (such as realistic group goals) create a productive work environment.

1. Pertinent examples in my organization:

    a. _____

    b. _____

    c. _____

2. Potential targets on my reporting staff:

    a. _____

    b. _____

    c. _____

3. Department targets within my organization:

    a. _____

    b. _____

    c. _____

4. Applicable enhancement strategies:

    a. _____

    b. _____

    c. _____

5. Notes:

☐ Jointly Established Motivators

1. Appreciation Techniques
2. Expectations/Outcomes
3. Future Objectives
4. Mutual Benefit
5. Pride
6. Professional Development
7. Work Ethic
8. Work Norms
9. Workplace Interaction

☐ Jointly Established Motivators

Appreciation Techniques: Methods are employed by which the organization and respective managers show their gratitude to the employee for work output and dedication to providing high-quality health care service.

1. Pertinent examples in my organization:

   a. _____

   b. _____

   c. _____

2. Potential targets on my reporting staff:

   a. _____

   b. _____

   c. _____

3. Department targets within my organization:

   a. _____

   b. _____

   c. _____

4. Applicable enhancement strategies:

   a. _____

   b. _____

   c. _____

5. Notes:

☐ Jointly Established Motivators

Expectations/Outcomes: Short- and mid-range goals are established between the employee and managers whose purpose is to increase challenges and level of accomplishment.

1. Pertinent examples in my organization:

    a. _____

    b. _____

    c. _____

2. Potential targets on my reporting staff:

    a. _____

    b. _____

    c. _____

3. Department targets within my organization:

    a. _____

    b. _____

    c. _____

4. Applicable enhancement strategies:

    a. _____

    b. _____

    c. _____

5. Notes:

☐ Jointly Established Motivators

Future Objectives: Long-term plans and goals are set in which the employee will participate and gain technical knowledge and ongoing professional development as an integral member of the work group.

1. Pertinent examples in my organization:

   a. _____

   b. _____

   c. _____

2. Potential targets on my reporting staff:

   a. _____

   b. _____

   c. _____

3. Department targets within my organization:

   a. _____

   b. _____

   c. _____

4. Applicable enhancement strategies:

   a. _____

   b. _____

   c. _____

5. Notes:

☐ Jointly Established Motivators

Mutual Benefit: Goals and objectives are established that result in positive action that provides clear benefits to the organization, respective managers, and the employee.

1. Pertinent examples in my organization:

    a. _____

    b. _____

    c. _____

2. Potential targets on my reporting staff:

    a. _____

    b. _____

    c. _____

3. Department targets within my organization:

    a. _____

    b. _____

    c. _____

4. Applicable enhancement strategies:

    a. _____

    b. _____

    c. _____

5. Notes:

☐ Jointly Established Motivators

Pride: Groupwide interpersonal investment is evident in the workplace, as reflected by a commitment to group goal attainment and self-fulfillment from group achievement.

1. Pertinent examples in my organization:

   a. _____

   b. _____

   c. _____

2. Potential targets on my reporting staff:

   a. _____

   b. _____

   c. _____

3. Department targets within my organization:

   a. _____

   b. _____

   c. _____

4. Applicable enhancement strategies:

   a. _____

   b. _____

   c. _____

5. Notes:

☐ Jointly Established Motivators

Professional Development: Opportunities are identified and facilitated by management for the employee to increase job-related knowledge, technical acumen, and business prowess.

1. Pertinent examples in my organization:

   a. _____

   b. _____

   c. _____

2. Potential targets on my reporting staff:

   a. _____

   b. _____

   c. _____

3. Department targets within my organization:

   a. _____

   b. _____

   c. _____

4. Applicable enhancement strategies:

   a. _____

   b. _____

   c. _____

5. Notes:

☐ Jointly Established Motivators

Work Ethic: An application of effort is demanded by management from the employee on a daily basis; it includes practical application of dedication, desire for success, and determination to meet established goals.

1. Pertinent examples in my organization:

   a. _____

   b. _____

   c. _____

2. Potential targets on my reporting staff:

   a. _____

   b. _____

   c. _____

3. Department targets within my organization:

   a. _____

   b. _____

   c. _____

4. Applicable enhancement strategies:

   a. _____

   b. _____

   c. _____

5. Notes:

☐ Jointly Established Motivators

Work Norms: A daily pattern of work activity is regulated and administered by managers in the interest of maximizing workplace action and optimizing employee comfort and productivity.

1. Pertinent examples in my organization:

    a. _____

    b. _____

    c. _____

2. Potential targets on my reporting staff:

    a. _____

    b. _____

    c. _____

3. Department targets within my organization:

    a. _____

    b. _____

    c. _____

4. Applicable enhancement strategies:

    a. _____

    b. _____

    c. _____

5. Notes:

☐ Jointly Established Motivators

Workplace Interaction: Relative harmony is present within a given working environment, marked by a spirit of cooperation and cohesiveness; although personalities might differ, the group objective of premier health care service is shared.

1. Pertinent examples in my organization:

    a. _____

    b. _____

    c. _____

2. Potential targets on my reporting staff:

    a. _____

    b. _____

    c. _____

3. Department targets within my organization:

    a. _____

    b. _____

    c. _____

4. Applicable enhancement strategies:

    a. _____

    b. _____

    c. _____

5. Notes:

Progressive Human Resources Strategies

This appendix, which expands on material introduced in chapter 7, contains personnel development and employee/staff investment strategies that can be implemented at any level of the organization. Utilize these 20 strategies, as well as the 60 potential applications, to upgrade your approaches to progressive, value-driven management.

Figure D-1 illustrates how the planning work sheets in this appendix can be used by the health care manager.

Figure D-1. Sample Human Resources Planning Work Sheet

On-Site Education Programs

Overview: In addition to offering in-service training and development programs, many institutions have implemented on-site educational programs for employee personal and professional enrichment. Such programs increase long-term employee development as well as exemplify concern for employee growth.

Potential applications:
1. College-credit programs leading to various degrees
2. GED prep courses and continuing education programs
3. Licensing/accreditation professional programs

Specific applications in my organization:
1. "Reading is Fundamental" sessions cosponsored with Madison High School
2. Junior college courses on-site on Wednesday nights
3. Accreditation prep courses for new nurse aides

Key players for implementation:
1. Education Department
2. Associate Director of Nursing
3. Human Resources Director

Prospective advantages to my organization:
1. Complete literacy at all levels
2. Greater "organizational investment" (preparedness, employee relations)

☐ Personnel Development Strategies

1. Affirmative Action Program
2. CEO Top–Down Interaction
3. Employee Referral Recruitment
4. In-House Training and Development
5. Joint Task Force Operations
6. Language Skills Training
7. Mission Action Committees
8. Outplacement Programs
9. Structured Selection Systems
10. Wage Surveys

☐ Personnel Development Strategies

Affirmative Action Program

Overview: Aside from adhering to legal mandates and sociological imperatives, installing a sound affirmative action program is simply good business. It ensures that the organization's composition will accurately reflect the demographics of the customer community. Designing a set of realistic approaches to affirmative action objectives is intended to ensure fairness and a sense of justice in the workplace.

Potential applications:

1. Firm, on-the-record, affirmative action plan and policy
2. Comprehensive affirmative action training and development modules
3. Human resources strategies aimed at affirmative action objectives

Specific applications in my organization:

1. _____

2. _____

3. _____

Key players for implementation:

1. _____

2. _____

3. _____

Prospective advantages to my organization:

1. _____

2. _____

☐ Personnel Development Strategies

CEO Top–Down Interaction

Overview: The effect of executive interaction in enhancing employee allegiance to the organization and resolving key issues that have potential organizational impact cannot be overestimated. Without sacrificing the power inherent in the traditional "chain of command" in an organization, the top tier of management can be involved positively in individual employee situations.

Potential applications:

1. "Hot-line" number available for random input
2. "One-on-one" performance evaluation system, in which an employee's written review is signed by the reviewing manager and the manager's superior
3. "Lunch with the boss" meetings each month

Specific applications in my organization:

1. _____

2. _____

3. _____

Key players for implementation:

1. _____

2. _____

3. _____

Prospective advantages to my organization:

1. _____

2. _____

☐ Personnel Development Strategies

Employee Referral Recruitment

Overview: Prior to looking to outside resources to fill open staff positions, the organization not only should look at existing employees for promotion but also actively involve them in the search process. Effective employee referral programs generate qualified candidates in a cost-effective manner, engender employee confidence, and positively utilize an often-overlooked source.

Potential applications:

1. Quarterly fee paid to employee recruiter over the course of the recruited employee's first year of service
2. Open positions published in employee newsletter
3. Alternative, nonmonetary reward system for hired referrals (such as a day off)

Specific applications in my organization:

1. _____

2. _____

3. _____

Key players for implementation:

1. _____

2. _____

3. _____

Prospective advantages to my organization:

1. _____

2. _____

☐ Personnel Development Strategies

In-House Training and Development

Overview: A successful organization is only as strong as its individual components, notably its human resources. The oft-used term *bench strength* refers to the wealth of talent an organization has across its personnel line, principally in positions of specific expertise and/or management responsibility, that inherently demands top-quality training provided by the organization.

Potential applications:

1. Technical education specific to accreditation/licensing
2. Professional development training in management
3. General application training, for example, customer relations

Specific applications in my organization:

1. _____

2. _____

3. _____

Key players for implementation:

1. _____

2. _____

3. _____

Prospective advantages to my organization:

1. _____

2. _____

☐ Personnel Development Strategies

Joint Task Force Operations

Overview: With the advent of numerous challenges to health care organizations to provide new forms of services and a wide array of new customer/patient needs, the participation of various employees is vital to new program formation. Their participation in these endeavors increases breadth of vision, morale, and performance investment.

Potential applications:

1. Matrix management structures for key projects
2. Advisory committees on new employee relations/human resources programs
3. Short-term councils on vital organizational issues

Specific applications in my organization:

1. _____

2. _____

3. _____

Key players for implementation:

1. _____

2. _____

3. _____

Prospective advantages to my organization:

1. _____

2. _____

☐ Personnel Development Strategies

Language Skills Training

Overview: Approximately 70 languages other than English are used regularly in the United States and Canada, both in the workplace and in social settings. Language skills training has the dual benefit of helping the foreign-born employee and the foreign-born customer/patient for both of whom English may be a second language.

Potential applications:

1. English as a second language (ESL) education
2. Specific-immersion language training
3. Key-phrase mastery programs for all employees

Specific applications in my organization:

1. _____

2. _____

3. _____

Key players for implementation:

1. _____

2. _____

3. _____

Prospective advantages to my organization:

1. _____

2. _____

☐ Personnel Development Strategies

Mission Action Committees

Overview: For a mission statement, operational credo, or organizational ethics declaration to be meaningful, it must be supported and embraced by all members of the health care organization, not just those in the executive suite. A mission action committee enables support of the mission statement and practical guidance on how to reinforce its relevance.

Potential applications:

1. Employee participation in construction of mission statement
2. Development of realistic action criteria
3. Recognition measures of mission-supported action

Specific applications in my organization:

1. _____

2. _____

3. _____

Key players for implementation:

1. _____

2. _____

3. _____

Prospective advantages to my organization:

1. _____

2. _____

☐ Personnel Development Strategies

Outplacement Programs

Overview: Financial conditions, organizational "downsizing," and staff reconsolidation all raise the need for occasional layoffs and personnel reductions in order to preserve fiscal stability and human resources strength. If not handled professionally and expeditiously, these moves can undercut morale severely.

Potential applications:

1. Consultant-controlled group outplacement
2. Internally generated outplacement approaches
3. Individual outplacement counseling and redirection

Specific applications in my organization:

1. _____

2. _____

3. _____

Key players for implementation:

1. _____

2. _____

3. _____

Prospective advantages to my organization:

1. _____

2. _____

☐ Personnel Development Strategies

Structured Selection Systems

Overview: Even with the most sophisticated training and development tactics, the most bountiful compensation scheme or intricate performance evaluation programs cannot redress the liability of poor performance from an employee who never should have been hired. Targeted selection systems, founded on sound structure and solid criteria, are the cornerstone of productivity.

Potential applications:
1. Clear interview procedures for all levels
2. Sound criteria for evaluating candidate response
3. Adherence to structured selection guidelines

Specific applications in my organization:

1. _____

2. _____

3. _____

Key players for implementation:

1. _____

2. _____

3. _____

Prospective advantages to my organization:

1. _____

2. _____

☐ Personnel Development Strategies

Wage Surveys

Overview: Health care employees are eminently aware of what the competitive pay rate for their profession is in their local area and, in most cases, the national scale for their technical specialty. In that money is a key motivator and measure of expertise, the health care organization must keep abreast of wage and salary scales.

Potential applications:

1. Wage surveys conducted by the human resources department
2. Surveys conducted and published by associations
3. Pertinent information incorporated internally

Specific applications in my organization:

1. _____

2. _____

3. _____

Key players for implementation:

1. _____

2. _____

3. _____

Prospective advantages to my organization:

1. _____

2. _____

☐ Employee/Staff Investment Strategies

1. Alternative Benefit Programs
2. Bonus-Incentive Compensation
3. Employee Assistance Programs
4. Employee Newsletters
5. Employee Suggestion Systems
6. Internal Recruitment
7. On-Site Education Programs
8. Personnel Development Plans
9. Stress Management Programs
10. Third-Party Grievance Systems

☐ Employee/Staff Investment Strategies

Alternative Benefit Programs

Overview: In view of shrinking health care compensation dollars, the need for creative ways to reward employee performance is paramount. Aside from insurance and traditional benefits, alternative benefits should be provided whenever possible.

Potential applications:

1. Matching savings and pension programs
2. Employee meal programs and cafeteria plans
3. Tax preparation assistance and financial planning services

Specific applications in my organization:

1. _____

2. _____

3. _____

Key players for implementation:

1. _____

2. _____

3. _____

Prospective advantages to my organization:

1. _____

2. _____

☐ Employee/Staff Investment Strategies

Bonus-Incentive Compensation

Overview: Progressive businesses in a capitalistic society must strive to reward stellar employee performance in a manner that is equitable and reflective of outstanding contributions. The implementation of such programs, and the clear understanding of the mechanics and rewards of such a system, inspire optimum performance from all employees.

Potential applications:

1. Management-by-objective bonus schemes for all employees
2. Organizational performance shared bonuses
3. Department-specific bonus programs

Specific applications in my organization:

1. _____

2. _____

3. _____

Key players for implementation:

1. _____

2. _____

3. _____

Prospective advantages to my organization:

1. _____

2. _____

☐ Employee/Staff Investment Strategies

Employee Assistance Programs

Overview: Human resources are key to the progressive health care organization. They are also potentially the most volatile and most destructive to productivity and hardest to assess relative to quantitative outcomes and results. Accordingly, the health care organization must provide its employees with a capable component of counseling and other personal services.

Potential applications:

1. Crisis intervention counseling in all areas
2. Family/dependent counseling and resolution
3. Appropriate professional assistance provision

Specific applications in my organization:

1. _____

2. _____

3. _____

Key players for implementation:

1. _____

2. _____

3. _____

Prospective advantages to my organization:

1. _____

2. _____

☐ **Employee/Staff Investment Strategies**

Employee Newsletters

Overview: Acknowledged as being among the more subtle motivators, an employee's familiarity with an organization—its goals, objectives, and history—strengthens commitment to top performance. An effective employee newsletter can further encourage dedication, spark interest in activities, and heighten pride at all levels of the facility.

Potential applications:

1. Monthly employee newsletter with wide distribution (beyond the organization and through the community)
2. Editorial staff composed primarily of employees
3. "Highlight" features, for example, employee of the month

Specific applications in my organization:

1. _____

2. _____

3. _____

Key players for implementation:

1. _____

2. _____

3. _____

Prospective advantages to my organization:

1. _____

2. _____

☐ Employee/Staff Investment Strategies

Employee Suggestion Systems

Overview: No matter what style of power and influence is employed by an organization, all employees must be provided an opportunity to provide input on the facility's direction, specific programs, and perceived needs. Suggestion systems can provide an acceptable opportunity for valuable employee input.

Potential applications:

1. Suggestion boxes or other traditional devices
2. Employee-participative "quality circles"
3. Attitude surveys featuring specific calibration (tailored to the situation and the organization)

Specific applications in my organization:

1. _____

2. _____

3. _____

Key players for implementation:

1. _____

2. _____

3. _____

Prospective advantages to my organization:

1. _____

2. _____

☐ **Employee/Staff Investment Strategies**

Internal Recruitment

Overview: The strength of an organization lies in its ability to attract and retain sound, *long-term* human resources. Implicit in this requirement is the need to promote from within whenever possible, and give current employees every possible opportunity to apply for openings.

Potential applications:

1. Prominent posting system for open positions
2. Interdepartmental coordination of posting/publication
3. Sound system of application, review, and selection

Specific applications in my organization:

1. _____

2. _____

3. _____

Key players for implementation:

1. _____

2. _____

3. _____

Prospective advantages to my organization:

1. _____

2. _____

☐ Employee/Staff Investment Strategies

On-Site Educational Programs

Overview: In addition to offering in-service training and development programs, many institutions have implemented on-site educational programs for employee personal and professional enrichment. Such programs increase long-term employee development as well as exemplify concern for employee growth.

Potential applications:

1. College-credit programs leading to various degrees
2. GED prep courses and continuing education programs
3. Licensing/accreditation professional programs

Specific applications in my organization:

1. _____

2. _____

3. _____

Key players for implementation:

1. _____

2. _____

3. _____

Prospective advantages to my organization:

1. _____

2. _____

□ Employee/Staff Investment Organization

Personnel Development Plans

Overview: It is the responsibility of every supervisor, manager, and executive in a health care organization to review the performance, potential, and promotability of every employee assigned to his or her staff. In conjunction with the performance evaluation process, personnel development plans specify training activities and other development endeavors and chart long-term performance objectives.

Potential applications:

1. Organizationwide implementation of a formatted personnel development plan (PDP) system
2. Segments on PDP forms for employee input
3. Increased emphasis on performance enhancement

Specific applications in my organization:

1. _____

2. _____

3. _____

Key players for implementation:

1. _____

2. _____

3. _____

Prospective advantages to my organization:

1. _____

2. _____

☐ Employee/Staff Investment Strategies

Stress Management Programs

Overview: With the increased demands on all members of the health care organization to perform at high levels at all times, negative stress in the daily workplace becomes more and more prominent and potentially destructive. It is in the best interests of the individual employee, and ultimately the health care organization, to provide stress management programs for all members.

Potential applications:

1. Comprehensive stress education efforts
2. User-friendly availability of fitness programs
3. Access to specialized professional expertise/care

Specific applications in my organization:

1. _____

2. _____

3. _____

Key players for implementation:

1. _____

2. _____

3. _____

Prospective advantages to my organization:

1. _____

2. _____

☐ Employee/Staff Investment Strategies

Third-Party Grievance Systems

Overview: Despite the best intentions and most enlightened management approaches, disputes inevitably arise between employee and supervisor at all levels of a health care organization and relative to any number of issues. The progressive health care organization must ensure that appropriate systems are in place to handle valid complaints or conflicts.

Potential applications:

1. Skilled employee/labor relations specialist(s)
2. Opportunity to discuss grievance with appropriate executive
3. Intermanagement mentoring and review panels

Specific applications in my organization:

1. _____

2. _____

3. _____

Key players for implementation:

1. _____

2. _____

3. _____

Prospective advantages to my organization:

1. _____

2. _____

□ Appendix E

Progressive Business Strategies

This appendix contains 10 customer community strategies and 10 organizational business strategies for potential implementation in your organization. Review these ideas, as well as the 60 applications, for utilization in your approach to progressive health care management.

☐ Customer Community Strategies

1. Citizen Advisory Panels
2. Community Action Programs
3. Community-Based Recruitment Programs
4. Community Investment Programs
5. Customer/Patient Feedback Systems
6. Customer Service Award Programs
7. Health Information Publications
8. Mobile Health Services Units
9. Physician Business Relations
10. Progressive Marketing Strategies

□ Customer Community Strategies

Citizen Advisory Panels

Overview: Marketing firms use focus groups in designing and validating effective promotional tactics and key product components. In a similar vein, health care organizations can use citizen advisory panels to elicit guidance on issues affecting the customer community and the organization's surrounding environment.

Potential applications:

1. Facility construction projects that affect local traffic
2. Community-directed products and services
3. Introduction of new health care services

Specific applications in my organization:

1. _____

2. _____

3. _____

Key players for implementation:

1. _____

2. _____

3. _____

Prospective advantages to my organization:

1. _____

2. _____

☐ Customer Community Strategies

Community Action Programs

Overview: The most permanent marketing impact a health care organization can make is the lasting perception in the surrounding community that the facility is ready and able to meet the new challenges of health care provision as they relate specifically to its operating environment. Strong, well-received community action programs can heighten the institution's visibility and its credibility in the community.

Potential applications:

1. Ongoing presentation of local health fairs
2. Bilingual services and target-specific services
3. Standby emergency action programs

Specific applications in my organization:

1. _____

2. _____

3. _____

Key players for implementation:

1. _____

2. _____

3. _____

Prospective advantages to my organization:

1. _____

2. _____

☐ Customer Community Strategies

Community-Based Recruitment Programs

Overview: Community investment in a health care institution is increased significantly when the organization hires from the local community rather than "importing" human resources. As a continuous business practice, local recruiting reinforces the organization's presence as a "good corporate citizen."

Potential applications:

1. Posting notices of open positions in five tactical areas
2. Publishing job openings in community newspaper
3. Use of local media and school career days

Specific applications in my organization:

1. _____

2. _____

3. _____

Key players for implementation:

1. _____

2. _____

3. _____

Prospective advantages to my organization:

1. _____

2. _____

☐ Customer Community Strategies

Community Investment Programs

Overview: Most citizens believe that the local health care institution is a public trust, similar to a police force, school board, or other public institution. It is important for *all* health care providers to understand that their business communities have this expectation.

Potential applications:

1. Local employee purchase programs
2. Sponsorship of high-visibility community functions
3. Appropriate support of school activities

Specific applications in my organization:

1. _____

2. _____

3. _____

Key players for implementation:

1. _____

2. _____

3. _____

Prospective advantages to my organization:

1. _____

2. _____

☐ Customer Community Strategies

Customer/Patient Feedback Systems

Overview: A successful business knows its success lies not only with its comparison to competitors but with how it fulfills customer expectations. Methods should be implemented to garner critical feedback, analyze it, and act on it.

Potential applications:

1. Standard customer population surveys
2. Targeted research methods, such as exit interviews
3. Hot-line numbers, visitor surveys, and InfoCards

Specific applications in my organization:

1. _____

2. _____

3. _____

Key players for implementation:

1. _____

2. _____

3. _____

Prospective advantages to my organization:

1. _____

2. _____

☐ Customer Community Strategies

Customer Service Award Programs

Overview: Although most health care institutions emphasize the need for all employees to recognize that good customer relations is an intrinsic, vital part of their work role, it is equally important for the organization to recognize and reward stellar customer commitment. A comprehensive system must identify high standards of customer service and adjudicate rewards.

Potential applications:

1. Management and employee committee to set standards
2. Customer/patient and visitor participation
3. Well-publicized standards and rewards

Specific applications in my organization:

1. _____

2. _____

3. _____

Key players for implementation:

1. _____

2. _____

3. _____

Prospective advantages to my organization:

1. _____

2. _____

☐ Customer Community Strategies

Health Information Publications

Overview: As a public relations tool, pamphlets and other publications can effectively convey useful information about health care issues. Their regular distribution by the facility contributes to the perception that the institution is *the* capable care provider.

Potential applications:

1. Regular monthly "Health Beat"-type newsletter
2. Special informational bulletins on AIDS and other topics of interest
3. Periodic bulletins on new organizational assets

Specific applications in my organization:

1. _____

2. _____

3. _____

Key players for implementation:

1. _____

2. _____

3. _____

Prospective advantages to my organization:

1. _____

2. _____

☐ Customer Community Strategies

Mobile Health Services Units

Overview: Use of mobile health service units helps to bring the institution into the community—figuratively and literally. Increased visibility, a wider spectrum of user-friendly services, and a demonstrated ability to reach out to (and into) the community are all tangible returns on money invested in mobile units.

Potential applications:

1. Bloodmobiles and other traditional uses of mobile units
2. Units specifically designated for field testing
3. Helicopter/airlift operation and other high-tech mobile capabilities

Specific applications in my organization:

1. _____

2. _____

3. _____

Key players for implementation:

1. _____

2. _____

3. _____

Prospective advantages to my organization:

1. _____

2. _____

□ Customer Community Strategies

Physician Business Relations

Overview: Local physicians not only provide the core of a health care organization's professional medical staff, they also represent a wellspring of potential patient referrals and guidance in significant community activities. To fully utilize the strength of sound physician relations as a business asset, the organization must tap both its marketing and medical expertise.

Potential applications:

1. Physician referral programs and incentives
2. Practice assistance programs and services
3. Strategic interface systems between physician and institution, including management information system (MIS) support

Specific applications in my organization:

1. _____

2. _____

3. _____

Key players for implementation:

1. _____

2. _____

3. _____

Prospective advantages to my organization:

1. _____

2. _____

☐ Customer Community Strategies

Progressive Marketing Strategies

Overview: With the health care business community restructuring itself almost monthly, every opportunity to publicize the assets and abilities of a health care institution should be explored and used as positively as possible. Selecting the best provider is the wish of every prospective health care customer/patient.

Potential applications:

1. "Ask a Nurse" and other informational telephone lines
2. "60-minute services" in testing and vaccinations
3. Alternative delivery systems and "1-day" outpatient services

Specific applications in my organization:

1. _____

2. _____

3. _____

Key players for implementation:

1. _____

2. _____

3. _____

Prospective advantages to my organization:

1. _____

2. _____

☐ Organizational Business Strategies

1. Community Executive Action
2. Executive/Manager Management by Objective Programs
3. Executive/Manager Retreat Sessions
4. Executive Leadership Action
5. Interdepartmental "Show & Tell"
6. Mission-Objective Teams
7. Open-House Programs
8. Organizational Advantage Programs
9. Organizational Communication Tactics
10. Staff Development Planning Systems

☐ Organizational Business Strategies

Community Executive Action

Overview: As the most visible player in a public trust organization, the health care executive, as well as his or her reporting staff, must participate creditably in major community activities. Such action increases the positive emotional investment the community places in the organization, the network of community contacts needed for conducting business, and the executive's interpersonal skills.

Potential applications:

1. Participation in noncontroversial local politics
2. Leadership of significant community projects
3. Membership on boards of directors/trustees of community organizations

Specific applications in my organization:

1. _____

2. _____

3. _____

Key players for implementation:

1. _____

2. _____

3. _____

Prospective advantages to my organization:

1. _____

2. _____

☐ Organizational Business Strategies

Executive/Manager Management by Objective Programs

Overview: Set job descriptions and delineations of responsibilities are inadequate in reflecting the total scope of a line manager or executive's responsibilities and can lead to disparities when compensating for performance and organizational contribution. Management by objective systems must extend past simple goal establishment and incorporate *all* aspects of performance.

Potential applications:

1. Bilateral participation in goal establishment
2. "Values" section added to performance evaluation
3. Critical contribution/significant action section added to performance evaluation

Specific applications in my organization:

1. _____

2. _____

3. _____

Key players for implementation:

1. _____

2. _____

3. _____

Prospective advantages to my organization:

1. _____

2. _____

☐ Organizational Business Strategies

Executive/Manager Retreat Sessions

Overview: To ensure that its vision, direction, and action plans are fully understood and supported by all levels of the organization, progressive health care organizations traditionally sponsor retreats attended by key executives and line managers. Retreat sessions should facilitate direct assessment of organizational direction and set firm plans for attainment.

Potential applications:

1. Annual retreats to review and redefine direction
2. Quarterly retreats augmented with educational sessions
3. Ad hoc sessions for introspective planning

Specific applications in my organization:

1. _____

2. _____

3. _____

Key players for implementation:

1. _____

2. _____

3. _____

Prospective advantages to my organization:

1. _____

2. _____

☐ Organizational Business Strategies

Executive Leadership Action

Overview: The primary function of the top two tiers of a health care organization is to provide ongoing action-oriented leadership, particularly in times requiring critical contributions from all members of the organization. Proactive preparations and quick, decisive reactions are needed to progressively meet current health care challenges.

Potential applications:

1. Cohesive board composition and sound interrelationships
2. Competent crisis management and media relations skills
3. Clearly defined action plans and reaction roles

Specific applications in my organization:

1. _____

2. _____

3. _____

Key players for implementation:

1. _____

2. _____

3. _____

Prospective advantages to my organization:

1. _____

2. _____

☐ Organizational Business Strategies

Interdepartmental "Show and Tell"

Overview: The vital link between concept and action is communication, from the top of the organization to the lower ranks and—perhaps more important—in the reverse direction. Equally important is lateral communication not only between departments and sections that work closely together, but also between unrelated units with shared goals.

Potential applications:

1. Cross-departmental presentations at monthly meetings
2. Scheduled interchange meetings between departments
3. Cross-training and orientation presentations

Specific applications in my organization:

1. _____

2. _____

3. _____

Key players for implementation:

1. _____

2. _____

3. _____

Prospective advantages to my organization:

1. _____

2. _____

☐ Organizational Business Strategies

Mission-Objective Teams

Overview: Special circumstances and atypical challenges mandate fusions of specific technical expertise, managerial acumen, and an assortment of educated perceptions and suggestions. Utilizing various executive and managerial talent creatively can be invaluable in problem solving, conflict resolution, and progressive action planning and goal establishment.

Potential applications:

1. Review committees for employee benefits
2. Crisis management teams and budget reviewers
3. Discipline review teams/conflict mentors

Specific applications in my organization:

1. _____

2. _____

3. _____

Key players for implementation:

1. _____

2. _____

3. _____

Prospective advantages to my organization:

1. _____

2. _____

☐ Organizational Business Strategies

Open-House Programs

Overview: On-site contact with the health care facility is helpful not only in improving community relations and interest in the local community, but it also holds subtle potential as an asset in recruiting new employees and in motivating existing ones. In essence, "showing off" the facility can increase employee pride, organization presence, and community interest.

Potential applications:

1. Annual open house for all employees/citizens
2. Special open house for recruitment purposes
3. Department presentations of new equipment

Specific applications in my organization:

1. _____

2. _____

3. _____

Key players for implementation:

1. _____

2. _____

3. _____

Prospective advantages to my organization:

1. _____

2. _____

☐ Organizational Business Strategies

Organizational Advantage Programs

Overview: The current health care business settings require that successful entities constantly upgrade operations and constantly seek opportunities to present programs and services that emphasize the organization's commitment to stellar health care services. The organization's executive staff, in conjunction with all employees, must identify and present potential upgrades for consideration.

Potential applications:

1. Intergenerational day-care services
2. New approaches to parking and traffic control
3. "Smoke-Out" clinics and sponsorship of other special events

Specific applications in my organization:

1. _____

2. _____

3. _____

Key players for implementation:

1. _____

2. _____

3. _____

Prospective advantages to my organization:

1. _____

2. _____

☐ **Organizational Business Strategies**

Organizational Communication Tactics

Overview: Feeling a part of the "big picture"—that is, identifying with, believing in, and contributing tangibly to organizational objectives—is a powerful motivator and yields a significant return in employee work performance. Paramount to employee motivation is the proper transmission of important information on organizational direction and actions.

Potential applications:

1. Promotional piece on the overall scope of the organization
2. Formal, regularly published statements on major organizational activities and events
3. Informal but total, well-calibrated communication in community activities and ongoing business relations

Specific applications in my organization:

1. _____

2. _____

3. _____

Key players for implementation:

1. _____

2. _____

3. _____

Prospective advantages to my organization:

1. _____

2. _____

☐ Organizational Business Strategies

Staff Development Planning Systems

Overview: The continuous strategic planning undertaken by an organization must stretch beyond equipment and fixed resources and into the realm of human resources, most notably throughout the ranks of entry-, mid-, and upper-level management. A comprehensive system of personnel development planning not only charts "backup" positioning but critical development plans, staff's long-term potential, and performance values.

Potential applications:

1. Quantitative systems of promotability/potential
2. Comparative data for planning group and individual training and development activities
3. Clear-cut organizationwide personnel data

Specific applications in my organization:

1. _____

2. _____

3. _____

Key players for implementation:

1. _____

2. _____

3. _____

Prospective advantages to my organization:

1. _____

2. _____